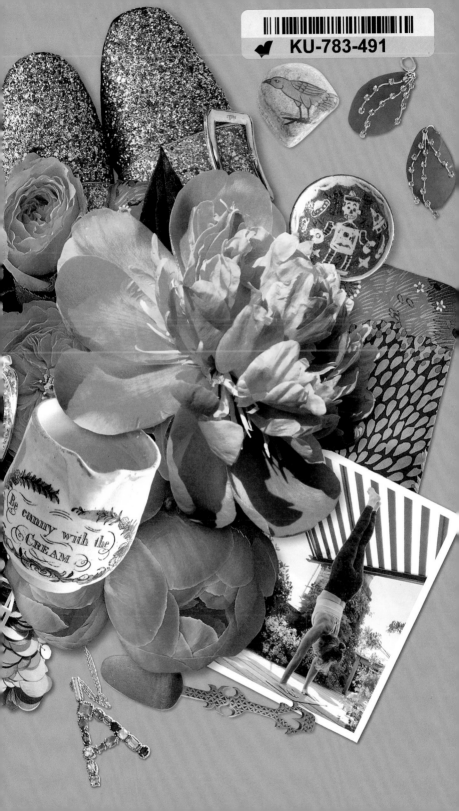

'Full of uplifting advice, practical wisdom and kind intelligence: I certainly felt more fabulous after reading it.' – Elizabeth Day

'A witty, warm, wise and illuminating guide to how to be your best self, inside and out. Deliciously upbeat and brimful of positivity, it's a perfect roadmap for the years ahead. I loved it.' – Mariella Frostrup

'Finally a book that challenges our tedious fixation with youth and turns the old rules about ageing upside down and inside out. With practical advice and spiritual insights, *Destination Fabulous* offers the kind of life-affirming guidance for womanhood I only wish I had known when I was 20.'
– Chioma Nnadi, vogue.com

'Anna Murphy joyfully reframes the gift of growing up, and older.' – Kenya Hunt

'A joyous celebration of the pleasures of growing older, and an empowering manifesto for changing our attitudes to age.' – Justine Picardie

Destination Fabulous

Dear Liz,

Enjoy your journey!

Anna x

Destination Fabulous

Finding your way to the best you yet

Anna Murphy

MITCHELL
BEAZLEY

First published in Great Britain in 2023 by Mitchell Beazley, an imprint of
Octopus Publishing Group Ltd
Carmelite House
50 Victoria Embankment
London EC4Y 0DZ
www.octopusbooks.co.uk

An Hachette UK Company
www.hachette.co.uk

Distributed in the US by
Hachette Book Group
1290 Avenue of the Americas
4th and 5th Floors
New York, NY 10104

Distributed in Canada by
Canadian Manda Group
664 Annette St.
Toronto, Ontario, Canada M6S 2C8

ISBN 978–1–78472–851–9

A CIP catalogue record for this book is available from the British Library.

Printed and bound in the United Kingdom

10 9 8 7 6 5 4 3 2 1

Typeset in 12/20pt Plantin MT Pro by Jouve (UK), Milton Keynes

This FSC® label means that materials used for
the product have been responsibly sourced.

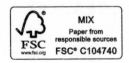

For Wendy, my pathfinder

M'illumino

d'immenso

Giuseppe Ungaretti

Contents

Contents

1

What's Gone Wrong, and How to Make It Right

Apparently there is something wrong with me. I am 50 and I am happier than I have ever been. Society tells us that the only way is down; that I am supposed to be feeling far less jolly than I used to. Yet instead I feel as if my life has been on the up for years, not necessarily in terms of my circumstances, but in terms of who I am, and how I live in and respond to the world.

I know, right? Obviously I am a weirdo. I have lines I didn't use to have, I have grey hair, but life has never felt better. Why? Well, first off, how could I possibly not be enjoying and embracing growing older, when being alive is infinitely preferable to the alternative? However, that's not all. The act of ageing has already opened my eyes to so much, and liberated me from so much, how can I not be continuing to find it an interesting – more than that, a compelling – ride?

It's not that I am getting everything right. It's not that I am perfect. It's not that I am remotely smug. The very opposite, in fact. I know there's more work to be done, always. But Anna at 50 is a better and more contented person than Anna at 20, 30 or 40. And I intend to be saying the same of myself now, looking back – I hope – from the vantage of 60, 70, 80 and beyond. Eighty-year-old Anna will be more than 50-year-old Anna. Yes, she will have more lines, and more – or possibly less! – grey hair, but she will also *be* more. That's the plan, anyway. And I am prepared to do the work, and to live my life in such a way as to make it the reality.

This is what *Destination Fabulous* is about. The idea that more, in terms of the years you have lived, can mean more in other ways too. I believe society is fundamentally wrong about ageing, and I hope this book is going to help you feel the same; to make you feel that the years you have ahead of you can be the best years yet. I also hope this book is going to turn you into a one-woman riposte to the misguided belief that getting older is a problem rather than an opportunity.

Certainly, ageing is a reality, so it surely makes sense to welcome it rather than fear it. *Destination Fabulous* is designed to be a road map that will lead you to become a personification of the truth – and it is a truth – that where you are right now, at this very moment, is exactly the perfect place for you to be. Its pages are nothing more than a beginning, a starting point, a place from which you can embark upon your own journey. The true path is for you to find.

After reading this book I hope that, like me, you will have found your way to the realisation that for you the future is all about becoming even more; about self-discovery, self-expansion, self-celebration.

I am not setting myself up to be an expert. I am a fashion journalist, not a guru. But I have always been motivated, both in my work and in my life more generally, to ask questions and to try to find answers. And I have always wanted to help women in whatever small way I can. I feel as if along the way I have picked up some things that might just do that, that might be worth sharing, from the practical (how to dress your best) to the existential (how to feel your best).

This book is my attempt to gather up the most useful and/or inspiring of my discoveries in one place. I am going to throw lots of ideas and suggestions at you. Not to mention a fair few gadgets that I have found to be game-changers. I also want to share with you some of the books I have come across that have illuminated for me truths around life in general and ageing in particular. Some of them you will know, some of them you may not. I have read them so you don't have to, but I suspect that you may well be encouraged to take a closer look at quite a few of them yourself. If the publication in question is not detailed in the text, more information is provided in the Notes section at the end of the book. Needless to say, when it comes to all of the above, feel free to pick and choose what resonates with you and ignore what doesn't.

It's not about impossible goals. It's not about running a marathon (unless you want it to be). It's not about denying the ageing process, nor attempting to erase its signs. It's not about letting everything go, either. It's about balance. It's about effortless effortfulness, or indeed effortful effortlessness. It's about keeping things natural and non-invasive. It's about the wonderment of the possible and of the present.

It's also about being more you than you have ever dared to be before. It's about going ahead and doing the things you want to do, even if other people tell you not to, or are shocked. In the last year alone, by way of two different examples, I have got the first fringe of my life, and the first younger boyfriend (only by five years!). Hilariously, people these days seem much more stressed at the idea of a fringe than a toy boy (please allow me to call him that), which seems like a definite move on to me. But anyway, suffice it to say, I am very happy about both.

As a journalist I have written about fashion, beauty and fitness for decades, so you can imagine some of the areas I will be covering in *Destination Fabulous*. However, be prepared also to be surprised. I know I have been! Twenty years ago mine was a conventional position on almost everything. Now I am not quite sure it is. Turns out I am a bit of a hippy, albeit one who still loves Prada shoes. When it comes to beauty, for example, I have learned a great deal from Traditional Chinese Medicine. As for finding your way to your happy weight, that point on the scale that makes you feel good about yourself and that you can maintain naturally, not through dieting, well, I now believe mindfulness is the missing ingredient.

Perhaps the most important thing I have learned when it comes to appearance is that looking your best self is, more than anything, about what is going on inside. The more fully realised you are, the more you find your purpose, the more that will shine out of you and the better you will look.

Panicked by how on earth to find your way towards self-realisation? Overwhelmed by the very idea of pinning down something as elusive as your purpose? Don't worry! This stuff is hard. That's why most of us haven't quite got round to it yet. And that's precisely one of the reasons why ageing is such a gift. Now you have enough years under your belt to start to know yourself. Now you have the perspective to begin to do due diligence on what works and what doesn't in terms of how you see yourself and the world.

What many people don't realise is that even the most long-held patterns of thinking can be changed if they aren't serving you, and that in changing them you can find your way to what is right for you now. I will share with you what has helped me to slough off my old skins and reveal the new.

As Jane Fonda, 85, said in her excellent TEDxWomen talk in 2011 (well worth a watch on YouTube), 'We need to revise how we think of ageing. The old paradigm was: You're born, you peak at midlife and you decline into decrepitude . . . . A more appropriate metaphor is a staircase. The upward ascension of the human spirit, bringing us into wisdom, wholeness and authenticity.' (Fonda's age, along with all the others I give throughout the book, is correct at time of going to press.)

The other day I was chatting with some girlfriends who are 20 or so years younger than me. One of them asked the group what age they would go back to if a magic wand could be waved. Immediately they started coming up with numbers. Twenty-one, said one. Twenty-five, said another. And so it went on. No one hesitated. Everyone had a number. Except for me, that is, the 50-year-old in their midst. Eventually they noticed that I had said nothing. 'What about you, Anna?' someone asked. 'There isn't any age I would go back to,' I said.

They looked, to a woman, amazed, if not disbelieving. 'Really?' they exclaimed. So I set about attempting to explain why I feel more content, more complete, than I have ever felt in my life, and that this is precisely because of being 50, not in spite of it.

Part of my answer was practical, and pertained particularly to the years that they were looking backwards at from their late-20-something and early-30-something perspectives. There was much that I enjoyed about both my teenage years and my twenties, I told them, but if I had to describe them generally I would say that anxiety was their primary characteristic.

There were the worries about whether I would pass my exams, get into the university I wanted to, land the job I wanted, find a flat I could afford, keep affording said flat, get the next job I wanted. This wasn't just superficial stuff: this was about attempting to find my place in the world. It was also about survival, or at least I felt it was at the time.

Then there was a deeper level of anxiety that pertained to people; that was yet more existential. I spent a lot of time worrying about what other people thought of me and attempting to find my tribe, be it friends I knew would properly have my back, or a partner who was as deserving of my love as I was of his. I suppose, if I had to sum it all up, what I wanted was to belong, even if I wasn't quite sure to whom or to what.

Now, at 50, I do belong. And I belong to the only person I can truly belong to: myself. I have learned the hard way – because the hard way seems to be the only way one can take on board the most important lessons in life, another reason why ageing has such value – that the most important relationship you can ever have is with yourself; that it doesn't matter what other people think of you, because only one person has the insight and knowledge to stand in judgement over you, and that is yours truly.

I have also learned that stressing never gets you

anywhere; that spending your present obsessing about the future and attempting to plan and/or control it is a waste of time. I now understand that living in the moment as much as possible is the only way to go, and that treating what life sends your way with as much lightness as you can, the negative as well as the positive, in turn lightens your load.

I have learned . . . well, so much. And I have learned it because I have lived 50 years, not 30, and because, somewhere along the line, I decided to become curious about this act of being alive, and of growing older, and to turn the kind of attention I used to give to passing those exams, getting that job, finding and keeping that boyfriend, towards me, and becoming better at being me. I realised that 'me' was not about any of the external accoutrements that I had been acculturated to think made up who I was, but about what I can only describe as my me-ness.

I was, I told my younger friends that afternoon, a far more developed person than I was when I was younger. Which meant that to go backwards to a younger age would be precisely that: a backwards step. Indeed my goal was to be yet more developed, 20 years from now, or 30 or 40 years, should I be given that blessing. Getting older was going to be interesting at the very least, I continued – another kind of challenge, another learning process – and life for me is all about keeping interested. I didn't even go there with the cliché that the opposite to growing old is, of course, dying.

By the time I had finished, my friends didn't look any less amazed, but they looked thrilled. And they wanted to know more. 'Really? Is that how 50 feels?' they asked. Did I genuinely not want to be younger than I was? Was I genuinely looking forward to growing older? Yes, yes and yes. They hadn't heard this before, they said. It made them feel differently about getting old; they, the unquestionably young, who were already wishing away years they had lived so that they could be younger.

Why do young women feel this way? Because society tells them that they should. For me one of the strangest and most counterproductive collective belief systems we have is the notion that ageing is bad, that it is to be feared. 'Anti-ageing' isn't anything other than a contradiction in terms. To be 'anti' something that is inescapable is bizarre, to say the least. To be 'anti' something that can bring with it great riches and newfound freedoms strikes me as just as odd.

Getting old is not without its challenges, but neither is being 12 or 22 or 32. We are often amnesiac about what we have lived through, partly no doubt because, with the benefit of hindsight, we think we could meet those challenges we once faced better. But even in that, the fallacy of such thinking is revealed. The benefit of hindsight. That's one of the many gifts that comes with living. That's what you have because you are 62 not 22.

I get where all this stuff comes from. It's a 20th-century cult that has profoundly changed the world. That was the period when a body shape akin to that of an adolescent male became the ideal for women; when women *en masse* began dyeing their hair; when teenagers were 'invented', and the kind of clothes that served as their signifiers, most notably jeans and trainers, became a new kind of uniform, whatever your age.

What are the origins of what has become almost

akin to a religion? Some argue that it was a response to socio-political instability; to war; to economic boom and bust. That may well be part of it. I think it's also to do with a profound shift whose origins lie in the Industrial Revolution that began two centuries earlier. Hierarchies were overthrown. It was no longer automatically the case that age and experience were best. Newness generally came to be seen as better than oldness. Change became more important than continuity and/or stasis.

There were fresh chances in life that weren't linked to age and experience or to class, but to youth and talent. That was, of course, a good thing, a very good thing, but we went too far, just as, previously, the talents of the young had often been overlooked in favour of the status quo. We took what could have been pure liberation and turned it into a different kind of straitjacket, one that places youth above age in the hierarchy, rather than alongside it, and one that dictates to everyone – but especially to women – that they fight ageing as an enemy rather than embrace it as a friend.

The Industrial Revolution also brought with it a

revolution in medicine, and with that came longer lifespans. There was no point worrying about looking young if you were likely to die at between 30 and 40 years old, as was the case in 1800. Indeed, if yours was a hand-to-mouth existence, as most people's was before the rise of the middle classes, there was no point worrying about anything other than that hand and that mouth, ensuring you had enough food to stay alive, and your other basic needs were met.

In the late 19th century, around 80 per cent of the British population was working class. Now around 58 per cent of us are definable as middle class. The middle classes typically have more bandwidth, both financial and cerebral, to think beyond the basic business of keeping themselves alive. They are the dream consumers.

So an entire industry grew up with the aim of selling them things they didn't necessarily need. The advertising industry that burgeoned in the 1950s and 1960s was predicated on creating desires we didn't know we had and selling us stuff – and concepts related to said stuff – that we didn't know we needed. One of those concepts was youth, which was a calling card for products as diverse as denim and hair dye. And advertisers worked hand in hand with the technology companies that were creating products that didn't used to exist in order to help us in our pursuit of what we didn't know we needed.

Dyeing your hair, for example, used to be a dangerous business. Should you attempt it, you might end up with no hair at all. It was also seen as shameful, a vainglorious attempt to fake youth – so much so that women who insisted upon going ahead would be hidden away behind a curtain at the salon so that they wouldn't be seen. When the chemistry behind dyeing was developed so as to be less perilous, Clairol swung into action with its now-famous slogan of 1956, 'Does she or doesn't she?' In the 1950s only 7 per cent of American women dyed their hair. Now Revlon estimates that it is 75 per cent.

The latest revolution is in so-called tweakments, designed to smooth the face of a grown-up who has lived life – and has the lines on their face to prove it – into that of an adolescent who is just starting out on the road to working out what it is to live. It is about rendering yourself a blank page. But who wants to be a blank page when you have so many stories to tell? For the moment, increasing numbers of women. The global facial injectables market was valued at $13.4 billion in 2020, and is only predicted to grow.

There is money to be made – a lot of money – in making us afraid to see lines on our faces and grey in our hair. Some of those younger friends to whom I was talking are already having injectables. I see the end results on the front row at the biannual fashion shows. Even if you have the best work done that money can buy, at some point your face may well end up looking frozen, swollen, misshapen and – ultimately – odd.

Of course the narratives around age have been in play since long before the last hundred years or so, especially when it comes to women. Fairy tales are populated with beauteous young maidens and dodgy old crones who are best avoided. But even the fairy tales didn't promise that age could be erased, and even the fairy tales didn't come up with something as macabre as the injection of toxins and the cutting of flesh in order theoretically to do so.

All of this is concerned with surfaces. Not what lies beneath. In obsessing over our lines we are inhibiting our ability to dig deep; to enjoy the here and now; to concentrate on expanding who we are. Growing older is a gift, an opportunity, not a disease. The women I admire who are older than me are the ones who are living their truth. It shines out of their every pore. Nothing has been erased. They are the most they have ever been precisely because they are no longer young, precisely because they have lived, and collected experience and wisdom in the process. And all of this is there to be read on their face.

None of which means we resign ourselves to the invisibility which is seen by many as synonymous with growing older. It's that idea of effortless effortfulness again. You aren't fighting your age, attempting to look or act like someone decades younger than you, because that is a fight you will ultimately lose. Yet neither are you giving up. You are keeping interested and interesting. This more than anything will transform the way you feel, and the way you are seen by others. And you are actively taking care of yourself, not just your spirit, but also the supposedly superficial aspects – face, body, wardrobe – that have an anything-but-superficial impact on the way you feel.

Because, yes, appearances do matter. In the last few years, I have come to understand more than ever the potency of clothes. Dressing yourself youthful, very different from dressing yourself young, is one of the simplest routes to changing the way the world perceives you. In *As You Like It*, William Shakespeare observed that 'All the world's a stage, / And all the men and women merely players.' Costumes determine how the audience views you; what role they imagine to be yours. It behoves you to dress for the part you want, not for the one that others want to give you. In particular, you don't want to be typecast, which is why – given the ageism around today – it becomes increasingly important as you grow older always to have something about your look that seems fresh, and ideally just that little bit surprising or attention-grabbing.

I am going to use that word 'balance' again. For me it's the key to life in general, but especially to ageing, not least because it is an active state that demands attention, and that can be lost the moment you take your eye off the ball. You don't look back or forwards. You don't try to fool yourself or anyone else that you are younger than you are, yet you maintain as much youthfulness as is possible.

There's a Japanese haiku I like that goes some way towards encapsulating how I feel about ageing:

Crisp autumn leaves
Rustle softly
Then blow away.

I don't want to be in denial. But I do want to rustle, rustle, rustle; to be dynamic; to be heard and seen. And I also want to be gentle, light, natural with it all; to rustle softly. Then when my moment comes I will blow away happily, having already rustled to my heart's content. An autumn leaf, lifted up into the skies. What a gorgeous image.

This book will share with you all the tricks I have picked up in my years of writing about fashion and beauty. It will tell you how to make the best of what you have got naturally. And much of it will go against the grain. There is so much you can do to lift and freshen your face, but the fact that it costs very little, and so doesn't make any company much money, means you probably haven't heard about it.

A lot of what we are told is plain nonsense. One of my most visible acts, for example, was the one I was most warned against: going grey. That may be the right choice for you, or it may not. Either way I am here to help every day be a good hair day from now on.

I hereby promise that by truly embracing who you are, by finding a purpose and a contentment that can be elusive to pin down when you are young, you will find your way to a new visibility, a visibility that is more potent than that which you may have enjoyed in earlier decades. Besides, that variety of visibility that a young woman often has can in truth be something of a burden. It is all too often transactional, an extrapolation of her sexual allure and putative availability. She is object, not subject. To be truly seen is to be truly heard; to be subject, not object.

If you age well – which isn't about erasing its signs, but about augmenting yourself in other ways; and, above all, about working on who you are, today, tomorrow and forever – you will find yourself more visible in the most encompassing sense of the word than you have ever been.

You will find 'you' as you have never found you before. And, always, *always*, there will be more to discover.

'Keep some room in your heart for the unimaginable,' the late Mary Oliver memorably advised in her poem 'Evidence'. Yes, that too. Always. *Always*.

2

Finding Your Purpose

Who are you? Why are you here? Who do you want to become? It's the root of all the trouble when it comes to talking and thinking about ageing that our starting point is our exterior, not our interior. We worry about what our faces are doing, and our bodies, and our hair.

Of course we do, because, as discussed, companies are making money out of us worrying about just that, and so they go out of their way to make sure that we are keeping on worrying.

And of course we do, because our physical appearance is what we see in the mirror every day. Our state of mind, our heart, our soul, don't greet us in the bathroom cabinet each morning. Although, tellingly, the health systems that pre-date conventional medicine, such as Traditional Chinese Medicine and Ayurveda, believe that the signs of all of the above are there to read on our face. In fact, we in the West have a more broad-brushstroke apprehension of something similar: we talk of someone looking heartbroken, for example.

Another reason that we focus on exteriors rather than on what lies beneath is that our interior life can be scary, especially if we aren't used to opening its doors and looking in its dark corners. Besides, surfaces are what we are told we can – should – change. When in truth the most important changes you can make when it comes to how you look actually stem from those you make within.

I am not saying that surfaces aren't important. How you present to the world does matter. Anyone who pretends that it doesn't is delusional. Not least because how you look also impacts upon the way you feel, the way you show up more generally.

Being in the best physical shape you can, and dressing to augment who you feel yourself to be, are for future chapters. We have plenty of time to talk about how to look the best you without spending lots of money or doing anything invasive.

What is for now is the real story, the only story that truly matters, and that's the story of what lies beneath. That, for me, has been the most significant discovery of my life. You can have what appears to be everything, and feel as if you have nothing. Conversely, you can have nothing, and feel blessed.

Contentment is a state of mind, nothing else. And getting older can bring you closer to embodying that way of being. You have earned perspective. You have earned the right to let go of what doesn't serve you, and to embrace what does.

As the Buddhist nun Robina Courtin says on her inspiring Instagram account @robinacourtin, 'Get old happily. Make the most of it. Your mind doesn't have shape, colour, or form, so it's not "getting older". Hopefully it's getting wiser. Identify more with your mind, rather than the body. If you want to pinpoint who we really are, it's the mind.'

I couldn't agree more. Just as significant for me in the last decade or so has been the discovery that you can rewire that mind, and thus, relatedly, change who you are at the most profound level. You don't have to remain fundamentally the same. With work, with patience, with presence, you can alter the things you don't like about yourself: open those doors; let the light into those dark corners.

Here is a truth that is largely missing from novels, films and television. Rare is the character who genuinely shifts, especially if it's for the better. That is because true change tends to be a subtle, lengthy process that isn't visible to the naked eye; that isn't necessarily discernible even to the person who has worked to change, until suddenly one day they notice that they are responding to an event or a person differently from how they once would. It doesn't make for a compelling drama, especially one that unfolds in a circumscribed timeframe.

This omission is also because the people who write our stories, our novels, films and television dramas, are human, as are the public figures who populate our screens and our heads. And the fact is that many humans don't do the work required to change, even the ones who are clever and insightful enough to write novels or run countries.

Yet there is another way to be, or rather to become. In his book *The Road Less Travelled* (1978), the psychiatrist M Scott Peck describes humans as mapmakers. We are at our busiest when we are young, he says, when we don't have much cartography to fall back on apart from other people's. The first map you draw is how to get your mother's attention when you are a baby. Sixteen years later it might be how to get the attention of someone you fancy that keeps your inner orienteerer occupied, or how to succeed at school.

Most people as they age get slower at making maps, and many come close to stopping. They just keep on using the old ones, whether they are still relevant or not. Peck's road less travelled is the one in which you never stop pathfinding, in which you remain just as engaged in finding new routes – and with them new experiences, new feelings, new learning – as the day you were born. As he puts it, 'Only a relative and fortunate few continue until the moment of death exploring the mystery of reality, ever enlarging and refining and redefining their understanding of the world and what is true.'

To combine the data you have accumulated over the years with a willingness to add new data and to reconfigure the old accordingly is one of the great gifts of age. It gives you the best of both worlds. You remain an adventurer but you now know the terrain, and if the terrain still surprises you – which it will – then you are better equipped to deal with those surprises. Ditto when the terrain changes altogether, which, again, as you approach your final decades, it may well.

In his book *The Changing Mind: A Neuroscientist's Guide to Ageing Well* (2020), the cognitive psychologist Daniel Levitin talks of a mode of thinking he calls 'generalisation', in which people use previous experience to find patterns and thus set up expectations. It's a generalisation that would, for example, lead you to believe that a spring day should be milder than a winter one. Though today, as I write – a hotwater bottle on my lap in April! – is a reminder that generalisations can trip you up, too.

The concept of generalisation is akin to Peck's

map-reading. And it's no surprise that scientific experiments have shown that older people tend to be better at it because they have had longer to draw up their maps. As Levitin writes, 'From a neurocognitive standpoint, wisdom is the ability to see patterns where others don't see them, to extract generalised common points from prior experience and use those to make predictions about what is likely to happen next.'

Of course older people are more adroit at that. Quite simply, they have more experiences to reference, and thus more complete maps. Yet the completeness of those maps can also be a problem; can lead you to overlook and/or eschew new turnings. And it is those new turnings that can animate your life until the day you die; can help you to find a purpose – or three – that you couldn't apprehend as clearly when you were younger and *everything* was a new turning.

The key is to maintain a kind of ambidextrousness that is mental rather than manual. How telling, indeed, that there isn't an equivalent term. It's about remaining consciously in the present, about path-making right here and now, while drawing on past knowledge, past thoroughfares as and when they are precisely relevant. It's about balancing generalisation with specificity and all the wonderment it can bring. It's about always being open to newness and to change; about remaining expansive and curious.

Indeed, I believe that with the right mindset we have a better chance at expansiveness than the young. We are hopefully no longer in survival mode, struggling to find a job, a home, a life partner, to have and raise a family. We have time, we have space and we can grow into both. Even that heightening awareness of the finite nature of life which tends to come with age can bring into fresh focus the importance of living as fully, as spaciously, as unguardedly as we can. We shouldn't fear death. We should use it to encourage us to live.

'Older adults' brains are plastic,' continues Levitin, 'capable of great feats of rewiring and adaptation . . . It's all about exercising your brain, pushing your brain in interesting ways . . . looking at the world differently, and then acting on it.' Or, as the 13th-century theologian Meister Eckhart put it, 'A vessel that grows as it is filled will never be full.'

Redrawing your maps is also about abandoning those routes that you inherited from other people. There is only one person who knows what is right for you, and that is you. Other people's maps have a tendency to be about them rather than you, or about someone else entirely, given that they too may have unwittingly inherited them. It can be difficult to apprehend what is yours and what isn't at any age, but it is nigh on impossible when you are a child, and not much easier when you are in your twenties and thirties. I believe you have the chance to get better at it as each decade goes by.

Parenting is all about the passing on of maps in ways that are at least as likely to be unhelpful as helpful. The Hoffman Process, a week-long residential multi-disciplinary therapy course, likens parenting to Chinese whispers, with one generation passing on to the next a distorted version of what has been passed on to them from the previous generation, who had in turn received it from the one before . . . And so it scrolls back *ad infinitum*.

Thus centuries-old preconceptions, their origins

long forgotten, can be kept unwittingly in a bloodline, despite the fact that they are serving no one. Hoffman's primary aim, it says, is to free children from their parents, and to help them set their children free from them. That week, which throws pretty much everything at you, therapeutically speaking, was one of the most fascinating – and freeing – experiences of my life.

A map can take the form of a story. Indeed, a map *is* a kind of story, and a story a kind of map. From the second we are born we are being told stories about the world in which we live and the place that we will have in it. All of which can, as I said, make it hard for us to work out even years later which are our stories and which are other people's.

One of the most pervasive stories in our culture is that we are what we have: that our baubles define us. Baubles don't take only the most obvious form of a designer handbag or an expensive car, of course. The face and the hair that many of us angst over as we get older are baubles. So too are our educational achievements; the house where we live; the job that we do. In Eastern philosophy even our most meaningful relationships are to some degree baubles, in that they too are another variety of impermanence, and can be shattered in a split second.

I think I perceived even as a child that the secret to life might not be about what you have, even though the bombardment of messaging was that it was absolutely about how many exams you *had*, what degree you *earned*, what job or husband you *got*, and so it went on.

The clue is in the language, as the German psychoanalyst and social psychologist Erich Fromm writes in *To Have or To Be?* (1976). He talks about the difference between 'a society centred around persons and one centred around things. The having orientation is characteristic of Western industrial society, in which greed for money, fame, and power has become the dominant theme of life.'

It's not that I was particularly motivated by money, and I certainly wasn't motivated by fame or power, and it's not that my parents were either. But such is the ubiquity of the having mode in our culture that it can be difficult even to apprehend the degree to which it is the water in which we all swim.

If you are a good girl, or boy, you do what you are supposed to do. You work towards having stuff, literal or metaphorical. For me it was about attaining garlands, first in education, then at work. And it was about ticking the boxes in my private life, too: a partner, a house. All in all it was, in the most precise sense, about being good: a good daughter, a good partner, a good employee. It was about getting my ducks in a row.

And it was only when some of my ducks wandered off, or were run over, or proved not to have been the right ducks for me in the first place, that I began to have an intimation that the equation I had been given for a successful life perhaps did not add up to the sum of its parts. Everything – everything – you have can be taken away from you. While what you are, on the other hand, can't be. It is you.

The greatest act of self-love is properly to come to know this 'you'. This you is the only person who is guaranteed to be with you until the day you die. To invest time in finding out who you actually are, what really matters to you, what you really want, is to give yourself the chance to identify what you need to add to your life, and what you need to take away.

Fromm urges us to 'accept the fact that nobody and nothing outside oneself [can] give meaning to life . . . [and] that this radical independence and no-thingness can become the condition for the fullest activity devoted to caring and sharing.'

Many of us spend our lives doing variations on the theme of our duty. Women in particular are programmed to put others first; to be a daughter, wife, mother, over and above being your true self. But how can you ever hope to find fulfilment if you exist primarily in relation to others? What hope have you of tapping into your unmediated you-ness?

I didn't even begin to start until the break-up of a long relationship when I was in my mid-thirties. At the time it felt like the worst thing that could have happened, but ultimately it proved the best. It forced me to look at myself: at what I was, and what I wasn't. It forced me to remake my life, and my mindset, in such a way as to suit me rather than someone else. How I feel about it now is best summed up by some more words from Mary

Oliver, this time from her poem 'The Uses of Sorrow'.
(Oliver's wisdom is a bit of a theme in this book.)

> Someone I loved
> once gave me a box full of darkness.
>
> It took me years to understand
> that this, too, was a gift.

The day that relationship ended was the day I began making a new map, my own map, for the first time.

What will give you meaning? What will give you joy? What will give your life a forward trajectory while also giving you pleasure and self-realisation in the moment? What will make you wake up each morning with the excitement of a child?

Is it a new passion, or an old one? Is it helping people? Is it a new job? Is it divesting yourself of people and patterns that don't serve you? Is it spending more time in nature, reading more poetry? Whatever, whichever, whoever. To stay interested is to stay interesting.

A mindfulness practice of some sort is a great way to

find your way to what your true self craves. So much has been written about meditation that this is not the place for me to cover the subject in depth. But I see the difference in myself when I practise daily versus when, as happens all too often, I let the practice lapse. With meditation comes detachment, and with detachment comes clarity and calm. And clarity and calm are a great starting point for anyone to gently interrogate themselves and their life.

These days, when I feel something negative, I am more able to step back from that feeling and explore exactly what it is and where it is coming from. Then I am able to acknowledge it fully, in order properly to let it go. When I was younger and I felt sad, I would become sadness, and it would become me. This made it difficult to process, and meant I had a tendency to get stuck in a particular state. Emotions are – as their name would suggest – supposed to be dynamic. You are supposed to move through them. If they become you, there is not enough differentiation to be able to do that. It's my meditation practice that has enabled me to find that differentiation.

You might be up for some self-growth in the most literal sense, perhaps reading books that help you understand yourself and your life better, or engaging in some variety of therapy. But self-growth can come by way of something else entirely. It can slip in through a side door: through a great friendship that makes you think and laugh; through a new hobby that challenges you and reveals new aspects of you. Everything – and indeed everyone – you add to your life from now on can and should bring the opportunity for self-growth.

Three years ago, for example, I decided that I wanted to be able to hold what's known as an unsupported handstand. A handstand in the middle of the room, in other words. The exact why's and wherefore's of this apparently peculiar aim aren't relevant here. Indeed, part of the value of the process for me is that this is a goal that isn't part of some wider objective, which would have been a given when I was younger, but an end in itself. What I will say is that I am a yoga practitioner, and two fairly new fellow yogi friends who are slightly older than me told me what joy they had found in learning how to handstand. 'It feels like flying,' one said. 'It's so liberating and empowering.' Some of my non-yogi friends think it is ridiculous. I couldn't care less. It's my goal, not theirs. All that matters is what I get out of it.

Mostly for me it still feels like falling, or failing. But occasionally I hold one long enough to get an intimation of what they are talking about. The handstand itself has become almost beside the point, because I have learned for the first time in my life true resilience, if not obstinacy, turning up day after day to try and fail at something for which I have no natural aptitude. And I have a new level of physical and mental discipline as a result. Learning handstand for me may not yet be about holding myself on my hands – sometimes I wonder if it ever will be! – but what it has given me as a person is inestimable. Handstand for me has become a purpose in my life.

Purpose is a big, grand-sounding word, is what I am trying to say, but it doesn't have to be a big, grand-sounding enterprise. Simply to live consistently in joy, in appreciation – which so few of us manage to do – is a remarkable achievement in and of itself. Simply to spread joy to others by way of whatever opportunities come our way each day, however apparently small, is to my mind the biggest purpose of all. It's that 'caring and sharing' referred to by Fromm, who also avers that we should make 'the full growth of oneself and of one's fellow beings the supreme goal of living'.

Growing older is our chance to transmogrify the thought patterns and behaviours that don't work for us any more, and possibly never did. It's our opportunity to find our way to what should surely be our ultimate purpose, which is to get better at the task of being human. Nothing big and bold is required, just better. Because, as the wonderful last lines of George Eliot's *Middlemarch* attest: 'The growing good of the world is partly dependent on unhistoric acts; and that things are not so ill with you and me as they might have been is half owing to the number who lived faithfully a hidden life, and rest in unvisited tombs.'

3

Saying Goodbye, Saying Hello

It's a commonplace in our culture to look at ageing as a diminution. Certainly you say goodbye to things: to the face you once had; to the body you once had; perhaps to ideas you used to hold about who you were or who you were going to become.

Yet why does saying goodbye have to be a bad thing? The Dalai Lama talks about cognitive reframing, a central tenet of Buddhism. Saying goodbye to what's old opens up the space for you to say hello to what's new. It is an act that can be an augmentation, an expansion, the very opposite of getting smaller. It can represent an existential spring-clean, when you can finally get rid of the dust, and move out some of that furniture you never liked in the first place.

Besides, if you are anything like me, you will be bidding farewell to much that is negative and that has never served you: to the insecurity of youth; the lack of confidence; to that tendency to watch yourself in the film of your own life as others might be watching you, rather than simply to live freely, without self-consciousness.

When I was young I often felt myself to be merely an object of other people's attentions, be that their expectations for me, their assumptions about me or the fact that they wanted something from me. (Or indeed didn't.) Like the majority of young women I also endured that most literal variety of objectification, the one that comes in the form of attentions from men I didn't know and/or wasn't interested in, and at – to make matters worse – times of the day when I had other things on my mind, and they should have had, too.

These days I am indubitably subject. I live my life for me, not for other people. And how transformative that is proving to be. When you define yourself primarily in relation to others, the danger is that the person who matters most – you – gets overlooked. Your needs and desires get lost and/or conflated with other people's. I am in no danger – finally – of doing that any more. The move from object to subject has been one of the most important farewells of my life, and out of it have come myriad hellos, the two inextricably linked.

In *Start Where You Are: How to Accept Yourself and Others* (1994) the Buddhist teacher Pema Chödrön says, 'Everything in our lives can wake us up or put us to sleep, and basically it's up to us to let it wake us up.' Saying goodbye to anything is the ultimate wake-up call.

Let's look a little more closely at the topic of the male gaze, because for me this is one of the most interesting goodbye-hellos around. People often talk about the invisibility that comes with growing older as a woman. In as much as that is the case – and I believe the way you act and dress can scupper this cliché along with many others – I would argue that with this supposed loss comes freedom.

Consider the nature of that youthful visibility, the degree to which it is predicated on your physicality, and by extension your sexuality, both of which can be treated as if they were public property, regardless of your thoughts on the matter. It's one thing to be found sexually interesting by someone you are interested in. It's another entirely to have other people's desires imprinted upon you when you don't want anything to do with them.

To be leered at and leched over is unpleasant. That is what being in your teens and twenties can entail, day after day, week after week. When we are living through it we experience it as a nuisance, a burden, an infringement, an assault. (Which, all too often, is precisely what it can become.) I remember experiencing it as akin to being looked at through a lens that excluded other more important parts of my picture. Notice how, with that idea of a camera, comes the notion of object rather than subject once again: someone else in charge of the composition, rather than me.

Why should we lament that kind of passing? And yet, as they age, many women do. They find themselves feeling wistful about the attention they once received. There's a great scene in April De Angelis' play *Jumpy* (2011) exploring just that, when 50-something Frances reminisces with her friend Hilary about being catcalled.

'I used to love that. Being a young woman being sexy on a bike.' 'You hated that, we both did,' counters Hilary. Frances says that she thought she hated it at the time, but now she misses it. She goes on to recount a recent night out in bar when she could feel herself receiving admiring glances from afar. 'This man my age, looked older, and not as attractive as me, OK, though, worth a punt, I could sense him at the edges of my force field being drawn in by my magnetism.' She decides to walk past him on the way to the loo. 'Thought I'd give him the full impact of my many charms at close quarters. I smiled, looked him straight in the eye. Dead. Not so much as a flicker. Total reptilian blank.'

What we miss is the ego-trip. Yet what age gives us, in this and so many other ways, is the opportunity to transcend so much of the nonsense that comes with ego. Frances doesn't particularly like this man. He is only 'OK', only 'worth a punt'. But her ego wants him to like her. What's more, we forget the grief that can come with this kind of attention. It is another example of those rose-tinted spectacles through which we are programmed to see being young.

We look back on our youth as all being good, rather than enacting a more honest appraisal, which would remind us that for almost every upside, there is a downside. Certainly there is some fun to be had when you are at your most sexually magnetic, but it is also limiting. You are more than the sum of your looks, not to mention your gender – or at least you should be – and when you are young you can be denied the opportunity to prove that fully.

Ours is a society which is, as discussed, far too focused on the superficial. Women in particular, however much we may resist the idea in theory, are brought to up to focus on how we look and – relatedly – our sexual desirability. It's hardly surprising. For centuries this was one of the only sources of power, and indeed means of survival, available to us. In *Jumpy* Frances isn't entirely joking when she quips, 'I've always thought of sexual attractiveness as an extreme fallback position. If I was starving.'

As you grow older you can be seen on your terms, not least because you know for yourself what those terms are; who you actually are. Far more importantly, you can be *heard,* if you choose to live expansively, truthfully, openly, loudly.

People like to put other people into boxes. It makes life easier in theory. It's hard to resist being put into a box when you are a young woman. As you grow older it can actually become easier to avoid being boxed up and stashed away. That is if you choose to age differently from the norm. To be non-conformist is to be seen.

In my experience the very things that you are warned against can be the very things that surface you like nothing else. Forget the idea of fading to grey, for example. Saying goodbye to my dark brown hair, and saying hello to my grey, has been one of the most attention-grabbing acts of my life to date.

I am also far more expressive now in my choice of clothes. I wear a lot of colour. I wear the kinds of things that a 50-year-old would never have worn a couple of generations ago. A fuchsia jumpsuit. Silver boots. A jacket with sequin flowers. Outsize jewellery and, as often as I can summon it, an outsize smile, highlighted with one of my favourite lipsticks. People call out to me happily several times a week. Men and women of all ages. This isn't catcalling. The energy is entirely different. It feels consensual. It feels celebratory. I am dressing to make myself happy. But what a pleasing byproduct that I should be making other people happy too.

Indeed, I would go as far as to say that I am more visible now than I have ever been before. And this is not just to do with my hair or clothes, of course, but the fact that I am confident in who I am, and what I think, and how I have chosen to live. That shines out of me. Of course I care about how I look, and I work at how I look, but I care far more about, and have worked far harder at, who I am. And that shines out of me, too.

When I turned 50 I wrote an article about my new visibility. In the same magazine there was an interview with Paulina Porizkova, once the highest-paid model in the world, and a few years older than me. 'I am now completely invisible,' she said. 'I walk into a party, I try to flirt with guys and they will just walk away from me mid-sentence to pursue someone 20 years younger.'

How could a woman who is so beautiful feel like this, when an ordinary-looking woman like me feels the opposite? Because, of course, hers has been a looks-driven existence. Her looks have been her job; more than that, her identity. The challenge that we all face as we age is to tune into our depths and become less concerned with our surfaces; to build a sense of self and of self-worth that isn't wrapped up with our appearance. That is perhaps yet more of a challenge for someone who looks like Porizkova.

As for those parties she talks about, these are the kind of parties that – and I know, because occasionally, as a fashion journalist, I am invited to similar events – are filled with people, men and women, who are more interested in transaction than in true connection.

What Porizkova may not yet realise is that she is saying goodbye to the kind of men who won't serve her, and who haven't in the past; men who are interested in her primarily for how she looks rather than who she is. In the same interview she referred to being treated as a 'trophy' by her ex-husband, the late musician Ric Ocasek of The Cars. 'When you are a treasured possession, as opposed to a person who is loved, you don't get to grow older. You have to stay the person they're obsessed with.' These are the men who are walking away from her at parties.

Porizkova is saying hello to the chance to forge a more fully realised version of herself, and find a place in the world that suits her better. 'The only way to gain visibility in our society is to look younger,' she says. I believe she is wrong, but she is only rehearsing what we are all told. Now she has the chance to find out her, not to mention our collective, mistake.

Did the artist Georgia O'Keeffe look young when she died at 98, in 1986? No. She looked remarkable, because she was remarkable; because of who she was and what she did, all of which was written in the many lines on her face.

In her book *Face Reading in Chinese Medicine* (2003) the late Lillian Bridges gives the example of the former American First Lady Eleanor Roosevelt as someone who looked better as an older woman; who grew into her face as she grew into her sense of self. Roosevelt was shy when she was young, and was considered to be plain. Side by side with a nondescript photograph of her in her twenties in Bridges' book is another of her towards the end of her life, when she had become a public figure celebrated for her insight and humour. In this later picture she is all sparkle, all charisma. She has many more lines on her face than she did as a younger woman, yet she is infinitely more attractive. 'Her personal essence shone outward from a less than perfect face,' is how Bridges puts it.

It's interesting to note, by way of another 'goodbye' that affects us all, that in Traditional Chinese Medicine, menopause – perhaps the ultimate instance of saying farewell – is seen primarily as a liberation for a woman. It is a phase when she shifts from one kind of creativity – the act of bearing and rearing children – to another, living more for herself and exploring her own interests and desires.

As Bridges writes, 'The ancient Taoists considered the time after menopause or andropause [the male equivalent, when testosterone levels drop] to be one of the most powerful times in life. When people had "Tamed the Dragon", which was a metaphor for ceasing menstruation or gaining mastery of the body's biological drives, the chance for enlightenment was significantly enhanced. This is because you are freed from your worldly obligations and are able to pursue your soul's work in accordance with your true nature.'

It is wonderful that menopause has finally become part of the public discourse in the West in recent years. Indeed, with all the books on the topic that have been published, it doesn't serve for me to cover it at length here. But what strikes me is that menopause is now so often written about as being synonymous with suffering and sadness; as being a bad thing; as being an experience that renders us victims. As Martha Hickey, professor of obstetrics and gynaecology at Melbourne University, argues in an article entitled 'Normalising Menopause' in the *British Medical Journal* (June 2022), media attention is turning a 'natural process into a narrowly defined disease requiring treatment'.

I believe we are also seeing yet another manifestation of our society's negative attitude towards ageing. Dr Max Pemberton, a practising GP, has written about his experiences treating women going through menopause. Although he says that hormones play an important part and is an advocate for HRT, he thinks it may be too simplistic to define these 'women's dissatisfaction with life and their sense of loss and malaise as a mere chemical reaction'.

It is at this stage in life, Pemberton argues, that the women he sees – 'so many I have lost count' – have the chance to take stock of their lives for the first time in decades. He writes that they 'have given the best years of their lives to other people – and now they're not sure why . . . So now what? For some women that question lays bare the huge sacrifices they have made – to ambition, status, income – in the service of other people.'

In a society that properly valued older women, and gave as much recognition to what they had achieved in their family life as in the outside world, the 'why' wouldn't be a question that needed to be asked, and the 'what' would come with an exciting, soul-enriching answer.

Katie Brindle, a Traditional Chinese Medicine practitioner working in the UK, tells me that menopause represents a shift in the balance of yin and yang in the body, the former a more passive, feminine energy, the latter active and masculine. 'The kidneys can be viewed as the batteries of our bodies. They inform the amount of energy available to us . . . and they oversee our overall ageing process. As we age, our kidney energy will naturally decline. Women begin to suffer with menopausal symptoms because of this natural decline and depletion of their kidney energy, leading to an instability in the yin/yang balance.'

The reason many women today 'suffer so much with menopausal symptoms is that they are simply not looking after their yin,' says Brindle, referencing our busy lives, which, given the degree to which we live in the world these days, rather than within the four walls of the family home, tend to be far more demanding than those of previous generations of women.

Aside from minimising stress and over-activity in your life more generally, Brindle advocates a range of techniques, from taking a 30-minute rest in the afternoon whenever possible – the time when, according to the Chinese clock, your kidneys are working at their hardest – to deep breathing in order to stimulate your parasympathetic nervous system or rest mode. She also recommends circulation-improving techniques such as *gua sha*, which is discussed in Chapter 5.

The silver-haired model Maye Musk, 74, not only has a jawline to make a 20-year-old jealous, she also has an attitude to life in general and growing older in particular that is inspiring. Recently I asked this former nutritionist and author of *A Woman Makes a Plan: Advice for a Lifetime of Adventure, Beauty and Success* about her thoughts on menopause.

'I had a dietitian practice for 45 years,' she told me. 'I helped hundreds of women with menopause. And I followed the principles that I taught my clients to get through it. You eat very carefully, become more active than you were, and you do fun things.' Fun things? 'You have to get your mind off the menopause. Everybody is terrified of it. I was terrified of it too! Because women would complain to me. But if you follow the principles then you get through it better.'

Of course, experiences vary enormously, and I myself have yet to experience the menopause. But of the myriad women I know who have, there are at least as many for whom it was comparatively unproblematic as for whom it was a big deal. And for everyone – whatever their experience of the nitty-gritty of menopause itself – there can be a newfound freedom once it is over.

Welcome to a life of still-white knickers, of not having to worry about getting pregnant or, indeed, not having to worry about not getting pregnant. Welcome to a life – most importantly – of time: time to dedicate to yourself. Welcome to a life when you also have the bandwidth to expand your love and attention further than perhaps you have been able to before, giving succour to more people, spreading your wisdom more widely. The so-called 'grandmother hypothesis' posits that, in contrast to other great apes, human females survive well past their reproductive prime because of the benefits that post-menopausal women offer to their grandchildren. You don't need to be a grandmother for that to be relevant, needless to say.

Of course, it may not be that you have much actual time for you just yet, with motherhood typically beginning later, and with the pressures of being the so-called sandwich generation, caring concurrently for children and parents. Yet the menopause is the sign that it is coming. An end is a beginning, always.

What I am saying, in short, is that it's time to re-evaluate what you are saying goodbye to, and embrace what you are saying hello to. I think it's a good idea to write a two-column list. One column comprises things you think are sad to say goodbye to; the column next to it is for you to come up with those hellos that you have the opportunity to welcome as a result.

Even something as apparently negative as physical decline provides an opportunity to learn. When you are young you can ignore your body, yet ignoring your body is a dangerous thing. As we age we are forced to check in with it more, and this gives us the chance to look after it more, and appreciate it more. It's also a chance to go within – to be, rather than to do – with all the potential for wisdom-garnering that comes with that.

Now it's time to write one more twinned list of those things you already knew you were happy to say goodbye to, the people and circumstances and stresses that never served you, and – just as importantly – those less appealing, not to mention less useful character traits that you have worked to divest yourself of. It will probably be easier to come up with the hellos that have followed as a result. Congratulate yourself on what you have achieved so far.

I mean, where to begin with myself in this regard? I used to be over-sensitive, judgemental and competitive, to name but three. Once I began to be honest with myself about these tendencies – which probably took me until my mid-thirties; no one could accuse me of being a fast learner – I could start noticing when they made themselves manifest, and work on unshackling myself.

I don't delude myself that they are done with. The phrase 'old habits die hard' is a cliché for a reason. Yet old habits can be dramatically diminished if you keep calling them into check. I am excited to see how much further mine can be dialled down in the years ahead. That, for me, is one of the many rewarding aspects of growing older.

The first half of your third and final double list should be – you guessed it – the work still to be done; the things you haven't yet waved off. It might take time to identify them, but once you have, the resultant hellos should come to mind more quickly. This is probably an endeavour that you will need to keep coming back to for a while, if not forever! Don't beat yourself up for the aspects of yourself that need improvement. Praise yourself for the perspicacity to identify them, and the bravery to take them on. Most people don't. That road less travelled of M Scott Peck's again.

Have you included in this a taking stock of the past more generally, by which I mean the people, places and periods of time that are no longer relevant to you? Nostalgia can be toxic, regret even more so. To live in the past is to fail to live in the present. To fail to live in the present is to inhibit your ability to experience, to grow, to love and be loved.

You can extract learning from what has happened to you, but don't dwell on what is passed, and also be prepared to recalibrate – and even throw out altogether – that learning if and when you ascertain that it no longer serves you. Your touchstone, your only touchstone, is the present.

'Accept – then act,' says the spiritual teacher Eckhart Tolle in *The Power of Now: A Guide to Spiritual Enlightenment* (1997). 'Whatever the present moment contains, accept it as if you have chosen it. Always work with it, not against it. Make it your friend and ally, not your enemy. This will miraculously transform your whole life.'

Mindfulness is, again, a great way to practise bringing your mind back to the here and now. I put off starting to meditate for years because I thought it was about not-thinking, and how on earth could I ever stop myself thinking? In fact, for most of us, meditation is about catching yourself thinking, then stopping and bringing yourself back to the moment, catching yourself thinking, then stopping again, *ad infinitum.*

It was the Buddha who first spoke of the 'monkey mind', or *kapicitta.* 'Just as a monkey swinging through the trees grabs one branch and lets it go only to seize another,' he said, 'so too, that which is called thought, mind or consciousness arises and disappears continually both day and night.'

The potency of meditation lies in the accumulation of stoppings, because that is what you can then deploy in your everyday life to bring yourself back over and again to the moment. The Buddha wanted us to aim for 'a mind like a forest deer'. I am worried that this might be too ambitious for me. I would settle for a slightly mellower variety of monkey. My research would suggest that the northern muriqui is the species to aim for. They spend a lot of time hugging, apparently.

Mindfulness is particularly helpful when it comes to disengaging from the stuff that all of us accumulate over the years: the sadness or anger when a relationship ends; the grief when someone dies; the fury at a perceived wrong, whether it's in your personal or professional life; the regrets about the things you should – or shouldn't – have done.

To be clear, it's important – always – to feel what you feel. To deny your emotional truth – how you actually feel about something beneath any layers of denial and/or conditioning around how you *should* feel about something – is to risk setting it in amber. But feelings should be dynamic. You should move through them, not stew in them for years. That metaphorical sofa that you used to like but is so uncomfortable that you haven't sat on it in a decade needs to go to make space for something else. So maybe bounce up and down on it a few last times for good measure, but then get rid. Now you have the opportunity to move in a new sofa, or maybe a love seat, or maybe – what the hell – a hot tub! Or maybe you can just enjoy the new-found spaacceeee.

There's a haiku by Mizuta Masahide, a 17th-century poet and Samurai, that sums things up perfectly:

My barn having burned down,
I can now see the moon.

What you should never say goodbye to, however, are those traits that are so often seen as youthful, even though many young people have nothing like them. Curiosity, enthusiasm, passion, optimism, openness. Trying to remain youthful in outlook is very different from struggling to stay young, not least because it is a battle you can win.

4

How (and Why) to Live in Joy

Many years ago someone asked me one of the most interesting questions I have ever heard. What single word would I use to describe my emotional resting state, the default headspace in which I dwelled the majority of my time? I knew immediately that, if I were honest with myself, I wasn't going to like the answer. I knew too that it was an answer that would surprise almost everyone who knew me.

The world saw me as a happy person. I was usually smiling, reliably upbeat. Underneath, however, I recognised myself to be something of a melancholic. My periods of true, heartful joyfulness – experienced within as opposed to performed without – were peaks in a landscape that was mainly low-altitude. It was just that – as far as everyone else was concerned – I made sure to look as if I had my hiking boots permanently on.

Alas, I knew that was simply how I was made, whether I liked it or not. Certainly I had the capacity for great joy, for huge enthusiasm, and I loved those moments when they hit. Yet to maintain that state consistently was too much effort for me; was not – oh the irony – my happy place.

Besides, surely to live joyfully day in day out in a world with so much suffering would be unthinking? Rose-tinted spectacles were all very well, but how clearly could you actually see through them? Surely they didn't help with perspicacity, with discernment?

The writers I loved most certainly agreed with me. Jane Austen may have given us happy-ever-after endings, but they came stitched on to a gimlet-eyed analysis of just how circumscribed the human condition – and, above all, the female condition – was during the Regency period. Two hundred years later, despite several revolutions, from the sexual to the technological, Sally Rooney isn't exploring the degree to which we have all been liberated from past strictures as much as how we have found new ones to add into the mix. Things have changed, but we have trapped ourselves in different ways. What is there to be joyous about?

So much! If there is one thing I have learned, it is that. And by recalibrating my responses to the world I have – to my stupefaction, quite frankly – changed my emotional resting place. I am not sure when it happened exactly. I don't think I noticed for a long time that it had. But a few years ago I became aware that melancholia is not my home screen any more.

How did I come to this realisation? On one occasion I checked in with myself, and I found that I was joyful for no particular reason; that I simply *was*. I checked in a few days later and – could this really be true? – I still was. And so it went on. I had rewired myself. I had – and I was amazed, and continue to be amazed by this fact – changed quite profoundly the daily Anna, which meant that the overarching me, the *echt* Anna, had become different too.

Of all the shifts that I have enacted in myself this, I would say, is the most significant, and is the one that has best equipped me for getting older. Life is a gift. I feel it these days more than I ever did when I was younger. Year by year I expand further into that awareness. Which means there is more of this abundance to come.

The Origins of You: How Childhood Shapes Later Life (2020) likens the study of human development to meteorology 'in that there are many factors and forces to consider that interact in complex ways over time and space'. The psychologists who wrote the book – Jay Belsky, Avshalom Caspi, Terrie E Moffitt and Richie Poulton – all worked on a research project set up in New Zealand in the 1970s that followed 1,037 children (to be precise) through childhood and adulthood, and encompassed speaking with family and friends as well as the subjects themselves.

We have – we are – a meteorological patterning, so the book's convincing thesis goes, one that can be changed by what it finds in its path as the years and decades unfold, but which remains a pattern all the same, with recognisable traits and tendencies. 'Humans have their hurricanes and rainy days, and bright, sunshiny ones,' the authors observe. Whether a storm becomes a hurricane, or whether a rain cloud makes way for sun depends on both the individual and on myriad external factors.

Which is why, as with the weather, attempting to predict someone's development over a lifetime is what the authors call 'a probabilistic science', one that obviates a 'one-to-one correspondence between would-be cause . . . and would-be consequence.' There is one key marker they identify, however. It is through resilience, above all else, that 'factors and forces that undermine human development can be prevented from working their black magic'.

What I would also argue is that we can decide to change our personal meteorology for ourselves. That we can focus on transmuting rain into sun wherever possible, or at the very least into a passing mizzle rather than a downpour. And that this should also be a goal because we are, in truth, not often best placed to distinguish inclement weather from clement in the long term. In the words of Herman Melville, 'Often ill comes from the good, as good from ill.'

It's not easy to tweak our in-person barometer, and the occasional frustratingly familiar squall may still cross your path - I know it does mine - but it can be done. Now I live joyfully. Which is not to say that I don't also still sometimes live sadly – not to mention tiredly, crossly, impatiently, stupidly and countless negatives besides. Yet my default headspace is a positive one. What happened? I relearned how to think, and I did so by relearning how to see and feel. 'Everyone thinks of changing the world,' Leo Tolstoy once wrote, 'but no one thinks of changing himself.' However, it can be done. Wonderment is all around us, every day, if we just show up and bear witness to it. If and when we do, our entire being shifts.

In his remarkable book *The Master and His Emissary: The Divided Brain and the Making of the Modern World* (2009), the psychiatrist Iain McGilchrist explores how the growing domination in recent centuries of the supposedly more rational left hemisphere over the more intuitive right hemisphere leads to 'the banishment of wonder; the triumph of the explicit, and, with it, mistrust of metaphor; alienation from the embodied world of the flesh, and a consequent cerebralisation of life and experience'. This is what we need to fight against in order to live in joy.

Let's forget the larger picture for a moment, and look at the smaller one. Let's take a cliché of poetry. The flower. Any flower. Really to look at a flower, to give it proper time and attention, is to be mesmerised by its beauty. And yet because our world is full of these stupendous floral entities, because they are a commonplace, we too often take them for granted.

Let's take something that doesn't abound in poetry. Our hands, for example. I am looking at mine now, as I type. More wonderment. The myriad ways they move, each of them impossibly intricate. The veins, carrying the blood that keeps me alive. The skin, such a mysterious entity, both permeable and impermeable. What a privilege it is to have hands, and to be able to use them. What miraculousness! There is nothing quotidian about hands, and yet we barely notice them most of the time.

Many of us are used to those moments of high-impact landscape, literal or metaphorical, that lift our spirits. It might be a mountain top. It might be a new love affair. It might be a joke that makes us laugh and laugh. It might be a conversation with a close friend in which we feel fully seen, heard, known. Yet we need also to recognise those smaller peaks that it can be all too easy to pass by without properly noticing.

There is a surrealism to reality, if we consciously bear witness to it, that can be reinvigorating. The other day my attention was caught by a strange shape in a distant tree. It didn't look like a bird. I couldn't work out if it was alive or not. What on earth was it? As I came closer I realised that it was indeed merely – merely! – a bird, particularly large, still and oddly shaped.

But that moment of failed recognition made me think about what a surreal thing a bird is. It sits nonchalantly on a branch. It appears to defy gravity with similar nonchalance, like a puppet without strings. Which led me in turn to think about gravity. What a weird and wonderful entity that is. Why, when one comes to think of it, must what goes up come down?

There is so much that we take for granted in our world, so much that is a kind of magic even when it can be explained by the laws of science, and so much more that can't yet be explained even by science.

The Russian literary critic Viktor Shklovsky wrote in his essay 'Art as Technique' (1917) of what he called 'habitualisation'. It is habitualisation, he said, that 'devours works, clothes, furniture, one's wife . . . art exists that one may recover the sensation of life; it exists to make one feel things, to make the stone stony.' In other words, the act of living can, through its repetitive nature, become desensitising; can stop you seeing, stop you feeling, stop you fully engaging in that very act of living itself. And art, among other things, can help to rescue you from that. His concept of defamiliarisation through art is a potent one.

Anyone who was lucky enough to visit Yayoi Kusama's 'Infinity Mirror Rooms' at Tate Modern in 2022–23, by way of just one example, will know exactly what Shklovsky is talking about. In the room subtitled 'Filled with the Brilliance of Life', the mirrored walls and the shallow pool of water reflect myriad tiny multi-coloured dots of light over and again amid the darkness. When you look at yourself in those mirrors you become part of that same pattern of light and dark.

Kusama (born 1929 and still working in her nineties) explains the thinking behind this work as follows: 'Our earth is only one polka dot among a million stars in the cosmos. When we obliterate our nature and body with polka dots, we become part of the unity of our environment.' We also experience pure, unmediated wonderment and joy.

Art isn't the only route to defamiliarisation, as I said. Simply to begin to check in with the wonderment that is all around us can begin to shift our emotional landscape. By truly seeing what is remarkable about the world in which we live, we can start to experience fully how remarkable it is to be here. To adopt the practice a few times a day of pausing truly to see something and register its incredibleness is to start to recalibrate how you think, which, in turn, will recalibrate how you are, which, in turn, will recalibrate who you are. It's my kind of pyramid scheme, the ultimate win-win.

Scientific experiments have revealed that not only do we smile when we feel happy, we also feel happy when we smile. You can fake it to make it, in other words. The act of smiling releases endorphins, which lift our mood and lower our stress. Thinking a positive thought sets in train a similar chain reaction. How you think shapes how you think.

And that is just the beginning. As the ancient Chinese philosopher Lao Tzu famously said, 'Watch your thoughts; they become words. Watch your words; they become actions. Watch your actions; they become habits. Watch your habits; they become character. Watch your character; it becomes your destiny.'

What Lao Tzu's statement makes manifest is the degree to which you engender yourself and, relatedly, the degree to which you can set about to change that self, for good or bad.

Personally, I had to develop a new lens through which to look at the world. Eventually that changed my character. Ultimately that change in character will be part of what shapes my destiny. You, in contrast, may not need a new lens. You may already be clear-sighted enough – not to mention full-hearted enough – to spend most of your time in joy and gratitude. But our society, which encourages us to be both goal-driven and, by extension, discontented with where we are in the present moment, doesn't make that easy. So you might, like me, need a few nudges to set you on the path.

If you do, I would recommend finding an easy way to remind yourself to come back to the moment; to feel at the very least gratitude and, whenever you can manage it, full-on wonderment. I suggest putting something around one wrist – a friendship bracelet perhaps, which, when it catches your eye, will remind you to stop and bear witness. You might like to rechristen it a noticing bracelet, and perhaps give it a little tug whenever it reminds you to bring yourself into the now, the better to seal the moment. A rubber band, some string or a few strands of thread would also do the trick. After a while, you won't need that prompt any more. The mental habit will have been formed. A noticing bracelet can be a useful way to help you change habits, too, be it reminding you to stand up straighter (one way immediately to look younger) or to soften your facial expression (ditto).

Even the most humdrum daily activities can be reinvented so as to be experienced differently. As Eckhart Tolle writes in *The Power of Now*, a book that is as potent an advocate for living in joy as it is for presence, 'If there is no joy, ease or lightness in what you are doing, it does not necessarily mean that you have to change *what* you are doing. It may be sufficient to change the *how* [Tolle's emphases]. "How" is always more important than "what" . . . Give your fullest attention to whatever the moment presents . . . As soon as you honour the present moment, all happiness and struggle dissolve, and life begins to flow with joy and ease.'

The most talked-about exploration of the power of positive thinking took the form of a controversial series of experiments carried out by the Japanese researcher Masaru Emoto in the 1990s. Emoto labelled different vials of water with different words, from the positive ('love', 'thank you', 'happiness') to the negative ('hate', 'I will kill you'). Then he used microscopic photography to capture an image of the water at the moment it began to freeze and form ice crystals. He suggested that the water labelled with love formed beautiful, regular crystals; the water labelled with hate formed ugly, irregular ones. Because Emoto's work was not peer-reviewed, his findings must be considered anecdotal, and they are certainly disputed. Dr Habib Sadeghi, a conventionally trained medic who now runs an integrative health centre in Los Angeles, is one medical professional who gives credence to his findings, however, and I have talked to others.

Let us remind ourselves that our bodies, once we reach adulthood, are made up of 80 per cent water. What label have you attached to your metaphorical vial? We have all learned from experience that what people tell us can change the way we feel for good or ill. We shouldn't be surprised that what we tell ourselves is yet more potent. To decide to live in joy and to frame your internal discourse accordingly is to set yourself on the path to doing just that.

A meditation practice will also help you to press pause; to see, and to celebrate. It will liberate you from the tyranny of thinking rather than just being. As Tim Parks writes in *Teach Us to Sit Still: A Sceptic's Search for Health and Healing* (2010), 'Morning thoughts rise like bubbles. I concentrate on the breath in my nostrils and on my lips. Only steady awareness of the body will still that mental fizz. I am not concerned when I don't succeed. The aim is quiet, but I will not crave it.'

Parks's book, as funny as it is insightful, is the perfect introduction to meditation for anyone who, like him – not to mention me – initially struggles with the whole fandango. It is thanks to an ongoing medical condition which conventional medicine cannot solve that Parks is forced to contemplate – pun intended – a mindfulness practice.

His entry point is so-called 'paradoxical relaxation', in which you lie down and calm yourself, then focus on some tension in the body without actively trying to relax it. In time, the thesis goes, the tension relaxes of its own accord.

To his disbelief, Parks – as determinedly sceptical as the subtitle of his book suggests – gradually finds his condition improves. By the final page, he is committed to daily meditation and credits it with dramatically changing his emotional state, both deepening and lightening it. (The realm of meditation is full of such paradoxes.)

'As words and thoughts are eased out of the mind,' he writes, 'so the self weakens. There is no narrative to feed it . . . Like ghosts, angels, gods, "self", it turns out, is an idea we invented, a story we tell ourselves. It needs language to survive. The words create meaning, the meaning purpose, the purpose narrative. But here, for a little while, there is no story; no rhetoric, no deceit. Here is silence and acceptance; the pleasure of space that need not be imbued with meaning. Intensely aware, of the flesh, the breath, the blood, consciousness allows the "I" to slip away.'

There are other, perhaps more tangible practices to cultivate. Seek out a passion or passions. It doesn't matter what. It just matters that it engages you, and makes you want to learn and do more. Adopt the attitude of an enthusiast, not only in this, but more generally. Be excitable. Be curious.

Roald Dahl wrote in his novel *My Uncle Oswald* of

'how important it was to be an enthusiast in life . . . If you are interested in something, no matter what it is, go at it full speed ahead. Embrace it with both arms, hug it, love it and above all become passionate about it. Lukewarm is no good.'

Lukewarm is no good. That's a mantra that works for me. To conjure in one's head – and in the heads of millions of others – rivers of chocolate and giant flying peaches, that's one way to stay in touch with one's inner child. Yet there are countless others.

As I write this, there is a 67-year-old woman in Hawaii, for example, who recently built herself her own skatepark in her back garden, a kind of plywood rollercoaster a few metres square. In the YouTube footage Jackie G exudes *joie de vivre*. She vibrates with happiness. She looks like a woman decades younger – not because she doesn't have lines (she does) or dyes her hair (she doesn't) – but because she is doing what she loves; because she is the opposite of tepid. 'As with every skatepark, the more you learn the bigger they get,' she says. 'This is going to get bigger for me.' The famous cellist Pablo Casals was coming from the same place when, in response to being asked why he still practised so much at the age of 80, he said, 'Because I want to get better!'

In one fascinating experiment conducted by a Harvard psychology professor in 1981, two separate groups of men in their seventies and eighties were taken back to their youth, or rather an ersatz version of it. In a secluded monastery near Boston a facsimile of the 1950s had been recreated, with Walter Cronkite on the TV, Cadillacs in the drive and Buddy Holly on the radio.

The first group to enter this strange time warp were told simply to relax, reminisce and enjoy themselves. The second group were told to immerse themselves more fully in the experience, to suspend disbelief and act as though they were their younger selves.

After only a week both groups showed a notable shift in their biomarkers. Everything from their sight to their skin elasticity, their systolic blood pressure to their flexibility had improved. The second group showed markedly greater improvements, however. Even their wrinkles had lessened. The men who had been told to act like younger men – to fake it to make it – had in fact become just that, as judged by scientific indicators. The conclusion of the professor who ran the experiments? 'Wherever you put your mind, your body will follow.'

So thinking and acting in a youthful way makes us youthful. That pyramid scheme again. Of course, living in your own variety of *The Truman Show* is neither doable nor desirable. The key is to find ways to achieve similar from a place of authenticity rather than via some kind of fiction or delusion. This comes by filling your life with people and activities that fire you up, mind and body. It's about remaining in explorer mode, the state in which you resided perforce when you were young and everything was still to be discovered. It's about maintaining that kind of curiosity that tends to be seen as childlike but shouldn't be. On the most profound level everything *is* still to be discovered, always. Who you are right here and right now is in permanent flux, and so is the world.

It's also about not trying to control outcomes; not overplanning. Explorers equip themselves as best they can, and travel wisely, but by definition they don't know the road ahead, and it would be delusional, if not dangerous, to behave as if they did. One of the most unhelpful teachings we receive when we are young is the idea that if we just plan hard enough, worry enough, stress enough, we can influence an outcome. That's wrong, of course. Getting older teaches you that, yet still we do it, because that is how we have been hardwired. It behoves us to do a spot of rewiring.

In *Start Where You Are*, Pema Chödrön, whom we met in Chapter 3, recalls one of the first Buddhist teachings she ever heard. 'The teacher said, "I don't know why you came here, but I want to tell you right now that the basis of this whole teaching is that you're never going to get everything together."' This was shocking for her to hear, she writes, and it shocked me when I first read it. We are taught that one day everything will be sorted. But, as Chödrön continues, 'There isn't going to be some precious future time when all the loose ends will be tied up.' What inhibits us, even imprisons us, is 'this continual searching for pleasure or security, searching for a little more comfortable situation, either at the domestic level or at the spiritual level or at the level of mental peace'.

To stop looking for more is to find more right here and now. It's another version of that idea of cognitive reframing to which the Dalai Lama refers. Besides, how can we know what the best outcome might be with regard to anything before we have even arrived at our destination? And how is carrying a heavy backpack of preconceptions going to help us get there in the first place?

When I think about what I lugged around with me, metaphorically speaking, until very recently, I have to laugh. My own expectations, many of them, in truth, other people's. The belief, for example, that the more I pushed and pulled, vaulted this pole and shimmied under that one, the better things would be.

Now I know that to travel light – and in the light – is going to lead me down the truest path for me, and that, just as importantly, I am going to enjoy myself much more in the process. Because enjoying yourself is what life is all about. Not in ways that are excessive or addictive. That's not your true self talking. Your true self might want a chunk or two of amazing chocolate, but it doesn't want three bars of the rubbish stuff. And your true self doesn't want you to loll around doing nothing all day either, I am afraid. Lukewarm is no good, remember?

We will be looking at how to tell the difference between what you may think you want and what you actually want in later chapters, learning how to check in with your true desires, be it around food, or sex, or whether you can face the Pilates studio again tomorrow morning. In the meantime it is simply important to acknowledge that your true self craves joy. And to recognise that the idea of living in joy – truly and unapologetically embracing a life engineered to make you happy – is a valid life goal, despite the fact that this is almost entirely missing as a legitimate ambition from many people's upbringing and education. No wonder it remains missing in action throughout many people's adult lives, too.

Luckily for us, we have reached one of the periods of life when we are best able to access that precious state, if we just allow ourselves to. The so-called U-curve of happiness is another example of the disconnect between the common narrative around ageing and the truth that many of us are living. It's in the final third of their lives that a lot of people find themselves happier than they were in the middle, the second half of the U curving upwards to levels they last experienced when they were young.

Here's one more potent hello-goodbye, if ever there was one, because it is the newfound awareness of mortality, of time running out, that makes people better able to live in the moment, and to spend those moments wisely, choosing more consciously what to spend them on and with whom.

When I first came across the idea of the U-curve a couple of decades ago I was delighted at the prospect. But gradually, as I read and thought more about what it means to be alive, as I began to practise yoga and to meditate, I realised that the U-curve wasn't enough for me. My aim was more of a J-curve, thank you very much. And that is the road I am on today, already a good few degrees higher up from the highest level of my youthful curve and, I hope, with a good deal more to come. My hiking boots are on pretty much permanently now, as I said. That's the altitude I am at.

It's not that I don't look back. I do. It's about balance, again. A little retro-gazing, not too much, is what serves. I use my past to help me navigate. I also use it as a way to celebrate who I am today. There is a Chinese saying that is usually described as a curse, an interesting duality in itself: 'May you live in interesting times.' Interesting times – responded to well – make for an interesting person. Without question it is the periods of my life that have been the most challenging from which I have learned the most. Were they a curse or a blessing? I would have said the former when they struck. Now I would say the latter.

Would I, at the time, have wished away my heartbreaks, my brushes with death, the occasions when work went wrong or friends let me down? Of course. But now I can see that they made me. Not immediately. Indeed, some of them broke me for a while. Yet ultimately, I didn't fracture, and that gave me a sense of wholeness, of strength, that I hadn't had previously. There's a widely loved Japanese haiku that for me sums this up:

> The moon in the water;
> Broken and broken again,
> Still it is there.

Then there is a Japanese practice known as *kintsugi* – 'golden joinery' – in which cracked porcelain is repaired with seams of gold so as to end up more beautiful than it was originally. With the help of passing time and growing consciousness, my breakings have made me better, made me more, brought me to a Now that is so much more expansive for me than my Then.

I have spoken already about the poems of Mary Oliver. There is so much joy in them. So much presence. She is all about seeing, really seeing, be it a blue iris, a charm of goldfinches, a small dog running in the snow, or indeed nothing much at all. Her poem 'Mindful' serves as a kind of credo, in which she proselytises for a life lived with full attention:

> to look, to listen,
>
> to lose myself
>
> inside this soft world –
>
> to instruct myself
>
> over and over
>
> in joy,
>
> and acclamation.

She advocates for finding that joy in even the smallest, most humdrum of things, in 'the prayers that are made / out of grass'. What a call to arms. Or rather, what a call to joy.

I only discovered Oliver a few years ago. Her oeuvre is determinedly glass half-full. She is a celebrator, not a commiserator. Working my way through *Devotions*, her selected works, I was blown away by her words, but I noticed that I kept double-checking them, and checking my response to them. I was looking, I came to realise, for naffness, for chocolate-box sentiment. My degree in English literature had, I eventually recognised, led me to believe that positivity equated to cheesiness.

I found some justification for my theory when I read Iain McGilchrist's *The Master and His Emissary*. Not only is it the right hemisphere where artistic endeavour originates, he writes, but it also has 'a tendency to melancholy . . . It is the right hemisphere of the brain that ensures we feel part of the whole. The more we are aware of and empathetically connected to whatever it is that exists apart from ourselves, the more we are likely to suffer.'

McGilchrist notes that 'music, like poetry, is intrinsically sad, and a survey of music from many parts of the world would bear that out – not, of course, that there is no joyful music, but that even such music often appears to be joy torn from the teeth of sadness, a sort of holiday of the minor key.'

This helps to explain why so many of our most celebrated writers, composers and artists tend towards a glass-half-empty outlook. It also sheds light on why, in the Western world, which for the moment largely rejects spirituality, we are so wary of anything that presumes to articulate faith and hope, meaning and goodness. Art can give us glimpses of joy, but given that much of it is 'joy torn from the teeth of sadness', we must also be committed to finding it for ourselves in our own world.

Can such an optimist as Oliver really be a great poet? Yes. She was awarded a Pulitzer Prize for a reason. Mary Oliver, who died in 2019, was that rare thing, a truly brilliant artist with a truly joy-filled outlook. Ours may be a world that tends to distrust positivity, that considers it facile, naive, yet this is another variety of programming that we must overcome.

Oliver's verse is suffused with belief; with the idea of life as a spiritual act. I have always considered myself an atheist, a rationalist, someone deeply distrustful of organised religion, with its patriarchy, and its exclusivity, its tendency to aver that some are in and some are out. Yet Oliver's beliefs aren't organised. Or at least, if they are, they are organised in the only way that seems to me to be true. As the 20th-century German theologian Albert Schweitzer once put it, the 'religion of love can exist without a world-ruling personality'.

We do need belief. Part of what has gone wrong in the modern world is that so many of us have lost our lodestar. Disappointed and disillusioned by the failures of organised religion, we have understandably given up believing anything. This may affect us more than we realise.

By way of just one recent example published in the *Journal of the American Medical Association*, researchers from the Harvard T H Chan School of Public Health and Brigham and Women's Hospital, both in Massachusetts, analysed almost 400 studies published between 2000 and 2022 that examined whether there was any link between spirituality and better physical and mental health, especially among patients being treated for serious illness. People who regularly attend religious services or describe themselves as spiritual tend to live longer, smoke and drink less, experience fewer symptoms of depression and engage in more physical activity, it was found.

Brought up to see a successful life as a series of achievements, the grander the better, we have lost sight of the power of being, and of seeing; of seeking out what and who gives us joy. Schweitzer was right. And so were The Beatles. All we need is love. That is the best religion of all. We need to love both others and ourselves. We need to love each day on this planet that we have been lucky enough to have bestowed upon us. We need to check in with the miracles of the natural world as much as we are able. We need to keep our eyes open for Oliver's 'prayers that are made out of grass'. As the 89-year-old Joan Bakewell said in an interview in 2022, 'There's nothing boring in the world. There's only a boring attitude.' It's not just writers who need 'to give the mundane its beautiful due', as the late John Updike once famously put it.

Growing older offers us the best chance we have to find our way back to love and to joy; to experience not just a U-curve of happiness but the J-curve. Lukewarm is no good.

5

Embracing Your Face

What does your face represent? It is the primary means by which you face – and the clue is in the language – the world. No wonder we give our face so much attention; everyone else does. No wonder, in a society that has so much anxiety around ageing, an anxiety fuelled by a highly profitable so-called anti-ageing industry, our face becomes our focus even more.

Women, in particular, are freighted with centuries of conditioning that encourages us to equate how we look with who we are. In fairy tales the beautiful are just that, inside as well as out. As the philosopher Heather Widdows writes in *Perfect Me* (2018), 'That we must continually strive for beauty is part of the logic of beauty as an ethical ideal.' To fail to meet the beauty standard – and in our society that standard is one of youthfulness – is framed as 'not a local or partial failure, but a failure of self'.

I am as capable as the next person of anatomising my face in the mirror, looking for all that has changed, which is a lot, and hanging on to what hasn't. But one of the many misapprehensions around our attitude to our face as we age is that we don't recognise the degree to which other people don't examine our face as we examine our own.

When you meet someone, be it a friend or a stranger, you don't scrutinise the detail. You take away a more generalised sense of how they look. And much of that is to do with how they are: whether they are happy, energetic, wholly present in the here and now, and, relatedly, wholly present to you, as you spend time with them. To appear joyful is not just an existential game-changer, as we explored in the last chapter. It is also the greatest beauty tonic out there.

There was one memorable afternoon on the Hoffman Process when I and the 20 or so other people who were on the course at the same time as me were led through a series of exercises that seemed more suited to young children. It all came across as ridiculously silly at first, not to mention confected. But eventually, one by one, at different speeds, we succumbed to the silliness. We started to enjoy ourselves. We larked around like kids. After a couple of hours we each had to sit and have a Polaroid taken of us. When my portrait appeared out of the mistiness I was amazed. I looked half my age. Everyone else experienced something similar.

Our face communicates our truth. As Coco Chanel once said, 'Nature gives you the face you have at 20. Life shapes the face you have at 30. But at 50 you get the face you deserve.' To work on any aspect of your character that needs working on, to process and release anything unhelpful that you are holding onto, that's going to work far better in terms of transforming how you look than the most expensive cream you can buy. That is not to say that there isn't plenty you can do to make your face look its best, be it with products or practices, and I will be sharing everything I have learned in this regard shortly. Yet to covet an unlined face, a face unmarked by the life you have lived, is not only delusional but damaging.

Delusional might seem like a strong word, but I stand by it. Here's why. In the UK the non-surgical cosmetics 'tweakments' market is currently worth £3 billion. Most users start in their thirties. Several times a year, thanks to my job, I sit on the front row alongside some of the most expensively tweaked faces around, barely a line among them. They don't look young. They look different. As they grow properly old, some begin to appear utterly 'other'.

For the first few years, when a woman is still young anyway, and if she is having what is called 'good work', there isn't necessarily a major disconnect. It may even be, with just the odd line here and there magically erased, that she looks a bit better than she might have done otherwise. Yet it always catches up with you. I have seen it happen over and again. And as a woman gets older, as the gap between the face she should have and the synthetic construction she has paid for in its place widens, she tends to look increasingly strange. As the onlooker, if you check in with your subconscious you will often find it worrying away at the wrongness, at what exactly it is that makes the resultant face not quite human.

An act that stems from vanity ends up damaging the very thing – in all its precious imperfect perfection – it was designed to safeguard. That is why, as much as anything else, it is vanity that stops me doing anything to my face. One form of injectables is designed to freeze muscles so – surprise, surprise – it can make you look frozen. Fillers fill so – surprise, surprise – they can make your face look plump in ways that also don't add up to looking natural. Anything more invasive can stretch and distort in ways that I for one don't want to be stretched and distorted.

The centenarian style icon Iris Apfel once told me she had made the same evaluation for herself. 'Unless God gave you a nose like Pinocchio's,' she said, 'why mess? You don't know how it is going to come out. Some very important people I know have ended up looking like a Picasso.'

As the psychotherapist Susie Orbach once observed

to me, 'When we see faces that are old but have had Botox, plastic surgery, they don't look any younger, they just look like they have done something.' Why do women sign up for it, then? 'Because of the current age compression at both ends of the scale, when six-year-olds are supposed to look like grown-ups and 70-year-olds are supposed to look 40.'

People also do it because an industry that, if it recruits you in your thirties, stands to make hundreds of pounds out of you every three to four months for decades is not honest about what the road map will be for the future. Say you start by just having a few injections between your eyebrows. That area of your face doesn't exist in isolation from the rest. What you do there has a knock-on effect on what happens elsewhere on your visage, which will in turn need more tweakments. If one area of your face is eerily smooth, this will draw attention to other bits that aren't. And when certain muscles start to atrophy, which is what happens when they are continually frozen, then other muscles are forced to work harder, causing more lines.

It's a brilliant business model, but not one that

serves the consumer. Sharon McGlinchey is a facialist with a wonderful range of natural products called MV Skintherapy. She once showed me only the top half of a couple of dozen Hollywood actresses' faces and asked me if I could tell the women apart. I couldn't. They all looked exactly the same. 'The area around the eyes is one of the main ways we identify someone,' she explained. 'If we change that in ourselves, we start to lose our identity.'

Not surprisingly, McGlinchey's approach to her own skin is entirely non-invasive, not least because she has had clients come to her with tear ducts permanently damaged by a muscle-freezing injectable (one has to wear goggles when she goes out, such is the sensitivity of her eyes) and others with filler that has moved out of its original position and then failed to dissolve, leaving a permanent ridge in the middle of the cheek.

Then there is what happens to your skin after years of 'successful' intervention. That aforementioned muscular atrophy will cause permanent drooping. Two individuals whose respective brands are built in part on administering muscle-freezing injectables recently told a beauty journalist friend of mine off the record that even they privately recommend stopping once you reach your sixties. What a terrifying prospect for someone who has been freezing their face for years. This is when you should switch exclusively to fillers, they continued. Yet the act of filling can create gaps within the dermis and, in turn, permanent indentations. Either way, someone reaches a point where they can't stop using injectables, even if they want to.

Beata Aleksandrowicz, another natural face expert who offers an intense variety of massage that lifts and lightens the face, says she has some clients who 'feel better and better' as they age. Others, however, 'panic. I had one client who was a beautiful woman, but she was under so much pressure not to have wrinkles that she decided to go for a facelift. When I saw her again she was someone I couldn't recognise any more. Her face had lost the natural asymmetry that created her character. She told me she regretted it. She had a lot of self-awareness. She told me she felt she had betrayed herself in allowing other people to tell her how she should look to be accepted.'

A number of Aleksandrowicz's clients come to her when they first abandon the injectables route. 'They are at that point when they are saying, "No, this is not who I am."' The way she tells it, this is a psychological journey, even a 'spiritual' one. 'If you have blocked any changes for years, denied that they exist, pretended you can be 20 forever, when you stop it can be hard. We want to be loved and accepted, and we have learned that to be loved and accepted we should have a wrinkle-free face. But your face is about much more than that.'

That's why I don't judge anyone for what they do to their face. What I do judge is our society for making us feel that wrinkle-free equates to lovable. Certainly I understand how it all starts. I was once invited to a flashy dinner full of rich, beautiful women. The rich tend to be considerably further down the road when it comes to facial interventions. Not everyone looked bad, but they all resided in a strange twilight zone of agelessness, anywhere between 30 and 60. Which, to be clear, didn't mean that they looked 30, or indeed 60, but like another species entirely. Nobody could smile fully, or raise an eyebrow, and I couldn't help but wonder if the more extreme cases had to sleep with their eyes open, as the 20th-century performer Liberace famously did.

My initial response was to reel at the kabuki-ness of the collective appearance of these women. Yet by the time I left I was wondering if I was unduly lined. Then I returned to my world where – by and large – women's faces move, and everything was fine again. Those women never leave this milieu, and a peculiar aesthetic becomes normalised, desirable; a prerequisite part of keeping up with the Joneses.

As this socio-cultural shift spreads further, and as our screens and our magazines are increasingly populated almost entirely by women who, if they are not young, and often even if they are, have faces that are synthetically adjusted, we are all at a version of that dinner party. Airbrushing is having a similarly insidious impact on our collective consciousness.

'On so many levels it is wrong,' said the actress Lesley Manville, 66, of plastic surgery in an interview in 2021. 'It feels like a betrayal of my sex. What are you going to do when you are 90 and looking 25? The message it gives to younger people is so awful, women of 24 are already Botoxing – where is that going to end? It's crazy. We get older, we die. You might as well embrace it.'

Or as another actress, Renee Zellweger, 53, puts it, 'There is a big difference between being your absolute best, most vibrant self and wanting to be what you're not. To be vibrant and beautiful you must embrace your age, otherwise you are living apologetically and to me that's not beautiful at all.'

And to quote one final actress – because, after all, who knows better about the scrutiny women face than an actress? – here's Helena Bonham Carter, 56: 'Collagen is not the only form of sexiness; there's character, fun, mischief and humour.' Hear, hear!

The most attractive older women I know have a face that is untouched, a heart that is open, a life that is full, a light that is on. Their faces are the books that tell the story of who they are and how they live, just as Coco Chanel observed. And there's something compelling about that when it's a life well lived.

As the late Australian psychologist Dorothy Rowe

wrote in *Time on Our Side: Growing in Wisdom, Not Growing Old* (1993), 'Youthful faces and figures can be very beautiful, but they are not very interesting. It is not until our face and body . . . reveal aspects of the life we have lived that our own individuality shines through.'

In Traditional Chinese Medicine, so-called face reading is used as a precise diagnostic tool. Those frown lines that so many people choose to erase, for example, reveal an imbalanced liver. In Chinese Medicine every organ has an emotional as well as a physical dimension. The liver processes toxins, but it is also where we store anger and frustration, toxins of another variety. Frown lines suggest the presence of all of the above.

I have frown lines myself. I would say they are one – two! – of the things I like least about my face. But I know what they are telling me. Sure enough, when I remember to relax my gaze, to be rather than to do, to slow down, my lines soften. Sometimes when I am on holiday they almost entirely disappear. Those lines are telling me something. I need to learn to tune in to what they are saying more consistently. I also need to learn to love them because it is then – in line with Tim Parks's aforementioned 'paradoxical relaxation' – that they will probably fade once and for all.

How can you ever hope to improve yourself, to move forward, if your face is frozen, a closed book forever more? Except that even a frozen face is telling us something. When does a face freeze naturally? When you experience fear and/or shock. What an irony that those women who embrace the cultural norm of fear around ageing by way of invasive work should make it permanently manifest on their faces.

When else does a face freeze? At the time of death. There are growing numbers of older women in the public eye whose faces look akin to death masks. And let's consider, while we are at it, the symbolism of injecting into the face a substance made from a toxin produced by the bacterium that causes botulism. Macabre doesn't even begin to cover it.

To fight is to fail. As Dr Habib Sadeghi writes in *Within: A Spiritual Awakening to Love & Weight Loss* (2013), 'Grass doesn't struggle to grow. Summer doesn't refuse to give way to autumn. Rivers always flow along the path of *least resistance*.' (His emphasis.)

Changing the way you live can change your face authentically, which in turn can make you look genuinely youthful. An inauthentic attempt at looking 'young', on the other hand, is, as you grow older, destined to fail.

I have a friend called Wendy who is in her late sixties and who – I don't know how else to put this – looks like a prettily wrapped present with a shiny bow on top. Everyone to whom I introduce her, whatever their age, immediately loves her. She has magnetism, even though she is a modest person, the very opposite of pushy.

Wendy once told me, in her usual self-effacing way, that she had become more attractive as she aged. I suppose I didn't really believe her at the time. Years later she showed me a picture of her in her twenties. She is right. She looks so much more now than she did then. It is not because she has had an easy life. Quite the reverse. Her husband died when her children were young, for example. It is the way she has responded to what has happened to her. In that instance, once she had managed to climb out of the depths of grief, she used her widowhood as a catalyst for a profound journey into who she was, and set about changing the aspects of herself that she didn't like. The face she has now is the face she has earned herself.

Chinese Medicine has a concept it calls 'peach luck'. It's manifested as a kind of magnetism, an energy that emanates from the eyes and is nothing to do with beauty as such. Peach luck is found in babies, their eyes twinkling with delight at being alive. Over time this energy becomes repressed in many people. Yet Chinese Medicine believes that peach luck can be cultivated by way of a life well lived; that you can actually develop more as you age. That's what Wendy has done.

I have already mentioned Lillian Bridges' fascinating book *Face Reading in Chinese Medicine*. If you are interested in learning more about exactly – and I mean exactly – what your face can tell you, this is the book for you. I can also recommend booking your own face reading session, either in person or over Zoom, with one of the graduates from her programme; mine was illuminating. (Look on lotusinstitute.com to find a practitioner near you.)

Bridges sums up brilliantly the problem with mainstream attitudes to ageing. 'Unfortunately we live in a world obsessed with staying young and beautiful,' she writes. 'This pursuit hampers the transformation of becoming timeless, which makes you beautiful in a way that transcends popular culture's standards. The glow that emerges from becoming your most creative self is easier to emanate when you are older and more spiritual. Only when you are comfortable with yourself can you become your most authentic self.'

The most youthful-seeming faces among the old belong to those who have retained a spirit of openness and curiosity, and who balance the wisdom they have gained from experience with a child-like joy in being alive. That there can indeed be a connection between interior and exterior beauty – as those childhood stories of princesses and evil stepmothers and happy-ever-afters led us to believe – is yet another of those paradoxes that populate the path of anyone trying to find their way to their best life. Who you are on the inside may not render you as young and beautiful as Snow White, but it can endow you with a magnetism, an attractiveness, that has a potency all its own.

Right, so that's enough about how the real work is to be done on the inside! How can we help our outside in the meantime? Again a dose of effortful effortlessness, or the opposite, will serve you well. Caring for your face isn't merely about putting cream on it, nor about paying someone to inject a toxin into it, or to slice it open and remake it. Caring for your face is about precisely that: giving it care and attention.

True care comes from a place of self-love as opposed to criticism. If, when you look at yourself in the mirror, you appreciate your face, rather than denigrate it, that is a great start. Don't concentrate on what you don't like about it. Focus instead on what you do.

What next? More important than anything is that you improve the blood supply to your face. It is blood that supplies oxygen and nutrients to the face, and it is blood that in turn takes away any toxins. So the single best thing you can do is massage your face, which will remove any tension, address congestion and promote lift.

My favourite tool to use for massage is *gua sha*, a plectrum of jade with which you gently yet firmly stroke the skin. If you buy only one thing I recommend in this book, it should be this. The best I have come across is Hayo'u Method's so-called Beauty Restorer. 'It draws blood gently towards the skin, increases microcirculation and boosts radiance,' explains Katie Brindle, Hayo'u Method's founder. 'The curved points can be used to activate specific acupressure points which will ensure good flow of *qi*.' (The concept of *qi* or *chi*, otherwise known as life force, the stronger and more free-flowing the better, lies at the heart of Chinese Medicine and its methodology for staying youthful.)

In the same range, I am also a fan of the Jade Precision Tool, which has a finer tip that is great for using on fine lines around the eyes and lips. I have even used it to remove age spots, a process that demands patience – it took me a couple of years – but that gets there in the end. Both tools come with instructions as to how best to use them.

Another way to improve circulation is through facial dry-skin brushing, which activates your lymphatic system, encourages trapped toxins to drain and exfoliates dead skin cells. I like the brushes of the facialist Alexandra Soveral: they come in a pair, and have just the right degree of firmness. A couple of minutes with these brushes and your skin is glowing.

Soveral has written a book called *Perfect Skin: Unlocking the Secrets* (2017), so you will be unsurprised to learn that she is something of a skin supergeek. She says that stress is one of the most damaging things for the skin. 'If your body is in the fight or flight state,' she explains, 'it withdraws blood from the skin and into the muscles in preparation for flight, which leaves your face with less oxygen and fewer vital nutrients.'

Soveral also regularly sees clients who just don't eat enough – especially fats – to nourish their skin. Dry skin lacks oil; dehydrated skin lacks water. 'From your mid-forties your skin doesn't produce as much collagen and elasticity. You need a two-pronged attack: to have enough protein and fatty acids in your diet, and to put the fatty acids on your skin in face oil form and massage them in.' Diet plays a huge part in your health and appearance generally, of course, and we will be looking at that in detail in Chapter 7.

Like many women I was initially wary about facial oils because I worried that they were going to make my skin look greasy. In fact it is only oils that have molecules small enough properly to penetrate into the dermis and feed the skin. Soveral's all-natural range of skincare – together with face massage and brushing as often as I can manage – has transformed my skin. I am a particular fan of her Angel Balm cleanser, a deep-pore cleanser that circumvents the need for extractions, which can cause permanently enlarged pores.

If your skin is dehydrated – telltale signs are dullness, under-eye circles and more noticeable fine lines – you need to make sure you are drinking enough water, turn off the heating at night and open the window a little, and avoid the kind of skin-resurfacing products that have become ubiquitous, from foaming cleansers to exfoliants. The hydrolipidic film that covers the skin's top layers acts as a barrier to prevent excess moisture from evaporating from the skin. Damage said film and you lose that moisture.

So much of what we are putting on our skin and doing to our skin is having the opposite effect to what we intend, fatally impacting upon its delicate chemical balance. Even products that pretend to be non-invasive can be problematic. The beauty industry bandies around terms such as 'natural' and 'organic' a great deal these days, but regulation is lax. It really behoves everyone to do the research before they buy and, when they find a brand they know they can trust, to stick to it. Small privately owned brands such as Soveral and MV Skintherapy tend to be more focused on quality and accountability and less interested in profit mark-ups than many of the big household names.

Another practice that I would like to pretend to you I do daily, but that if I am honest I properly manage a handful of times a week, is Carole Maggio's Facercise® programme, which has been recommended to me by experts as the best facial exercise programme around, and which can be downloaded or bought in book or DVD form. It includes around 13 simple – albeit slightly odd! – exercises aimed to lift and shape. My cheekbones in particular become noticeably more defined when I have been being good and sticking to a regular routine.

Some more gadgets that work. The most peculiar is a contraption called a Patakara, which was invented by a Japanese professor at a medical and dental college in Tokyo. It was recommended to me for reducing jaw tension; I was grinding my teeth at night. Imagine something that looks a bit like a baby's dummy, but which is sprung, so that you have to hold your mouth actively closed for it not to drop out. The idea is that you use it for up to 15 minutes a day to exercise both your mouth and facial muscles. I know. Weird. However, after a few weeks' of use I noticed, as the website promises, that my face had started to lift.

One more bit of Eastern otherness that comes close in terms of peculiarity is a *chi* machine, otherwise known as a passive exerciser. I would go as far as to say that mine has changed my life. I was first told about *chi* machines by a yoga teacher many years ago, at a time when I was still sceptical at best – if not outright scoffing – at the very idea of *chi*, never mind a machine that might stimulate it. *Chi* is, as discussed, the name Chinese Medicine gives to life force. In Ayurveda it is known as *prana*.

A simple illustration of what *chi* means is to imagine a person lying in bed who is alive one minute, then passes into death the next. In those first few moments of death they may, with the exception of their chest no longer rising and falling as they breathe, appear exactly the same as they did in their last few minutes of life. All that is missing, as yet indiscernible to the eye, is their *chi*.

Disciplines such as t'ai chi, chi gong and yoga are all different methodologies for increasing and controlling *chi*. A *chi* machine is a shortcut, if you will, a cheat. Or perhaps it would be more accurate to call it a *chi*-eat! It's the size of a couple of shoe boxes, and has two rowlock-like attachments. You lie on the floor, put your ankles in the rowlocks, switch the machine on and those rowlocks move from side to side, slowly shaking any tension out of your body and making you feel both relaxed and invigorated. If you are lucky, after a session of five to ten minutes you may experience a twinkling, sparkling surge of *chi* running up and down your body.

That comes and goes. It isn't to be relied upon. But what I have found to be a constant during my years of use is that my face looks much lighter and brighter when I am using it regularly. The *chi* machine is also great for reducing tension in the body, and I have even found that it can quite literally shake stress and emotional upset out of the body. Mine has helped me get through a couple of upheavals in both my professional and my private life.

I also rate Hayo'u Method's Clear Quartz Crystal Eye Mask, which releases tension in the eye area and decreases puffiness. Then there's the Light Salon's Boost LED Face Mask, which – like the *chi* machine – is another proper investment, but truly impactful when it comes to reducing the appearance of wrinkles, improving hydration and evening out skin tone.

I am not even going to try to claim to you that I am as consistent with all of the above as I should be. I am human! Very human! It's easy to skip one or two (or three or four) things, when you are tired and/or life is busy. (And when aren't you? And when isn't it?) I don't beat myself up when I let things drop, but I always try to find my way back again. Because I know this stuff works. And because, even more importantly, I know I am worth it.

Once your skin is in good condition I believe that the best thing you can do when it comes to make-up is leave it largely alone. I use under-eye concealer, and I cover up any blemishes, but otherwise my skin is bare. What I always do, however, is add something into the mix that is genre-busting, usually a popping lipstick (I find a matte or demi-matte more youthful-looking), or occasionally a similarly strong eyeliner, never both at once.

One of my favourite sources of inspiration for older style is the Instagram account @and.bloom, and the resultant book *And Bloom: The Art of Ageing Unapologetically* (2021). It's the work of the Dutch photographer and stylist Denise Boomkens, who is in her late forties and who styles and shoots older women to look their most fabulous.

Boomkens' approach to make-up is exactly the same as mine. 'The classic approach to make-up, with foundation and powder, doesn't work when you are older,' she tells me. 'It gets into your wrinkles.' Like me she favours lips and/or eyes that ping with the kind of colour that most older women would probably eschew at first glance. 'I think it's really good to have an accent,' she explains. 'A bright lipstick or eyeliner with otherwise natural make-up works very well.'

Usually my signature flourish is my lipstick. My favourites are matte brights from MAC Cosmetics: Lady Danger (an orange-red), Relentlessly Red (a pink-red), Style Shocked! (a hot orange) and Candy Yum-Yum (a hot pink). I have lost count of the number of readers of my column who have got in touch over the years to tell me how much one of those lipsticks has changed the way they look and feel.

On the occasions when I accent my eyes, I favour Sisley's Phyto Eye-Twist, with a chunky tip that puts it somewhere between an eye pencil and a shadow, perhaps Lagoon (a turquoise blue), Emerald (no prizes for what shade that is!) or Amethyst (ditto!). For a finer line, try Chanel's Stylo Yeux, which comes in an especially good range of colours that somehow manage to be both stealth and punch. (Prune and Rose Cuivré are my two go-tos.) I always wear mascara, and I am evangelical about both Revitalash and Revitabrow, which may be expensive products but – if you are dealing with sparse eyelashes or eyebrows – will transform the natural framing of your eyes.

Boomkens herself is a former model, and looks ravishing. How, natural beauty that she is, can she claim insight into what ageing is like for others? 'Not all the women I photograph are beautiful,' she says. 'Not all of them have a jawline. But every woman has something beautiful about her – her grey hair, her red lips. It's that "something beautiful" that I set out to highlight in my pictures.'

The more we highlight our own internal 'something beautiful', the better we will face the world.

6

How to Have a Good Hair Day
Every Day

When, just under a decade ago, I started to tell people that I was thinking about stopping dyeing my hair, they were horrified. I was in my early forties. I had started going grey in my mid-thirties; early, like my mother before me. My family and my then partner were encouraging, but everyone else seemed to think it would be a disastrous act. I would appear so much older! I would be overlooked at work! I would look as if I had given up! I would become invisible! I can't pretend that I wasn't a little unnerved. But I went ahead anyway.

Today I can say without question that the act of embracing my natural hair colour has proved my most hi-vis move of recent years, possibly of my entire life. At least a couple of times a week these days I am congratulated on my hair by strangers of every age, men and women. It's young men and women who most often comment, be it on the street, in a shop or restaurant, or on public transport.

I am not alone in this new-found visibility. When, at 60, Maye Musk first embraced her now-signature silver barnet, she told me, 'I remember the agent I was with at the time said, "We can't send you out like that. Nobody will book you."' Wrong! Suddenly she was a magazine covergirl. (Girl?! Even the terminology is telling.) Then there was a giant rendering of her on a billboard in Times Square in New York. At an age when many women are lamenting their supposed invisibility she says she is 'way, *way* more visible than I have ever been before'. One chapter in her book is entitled 'Silver is the New Blond'.

I was surprised by the impact my transformation had, I must admit, although I am still waiting to be booked for my own billboard! I hadn't factored in, back when I was considering making the change, the degree to which grey hair was becoming fashionable; that #grannyhair had become a thing on social media, and that women half my age were faking a version of what I could pull off naturally.

It was the male attention that most caught me off guard, however. I had originally wondered whether I would be brave enough to stop dyeing if I hadn't had a partner at the time. When I eventually ended that relationship I was perfectly placed to find out whether those fears of mine had been justified. And I can report that they weren't.

When I joined the dating apps, the aspect of my appearance that I was complimented on more than anything else was my hair. I am sure there were men who didn't like it, of course, just as there were men who weren't drawn to other aspects of the way I look or indeed what I said. But that's normal. And that doesn't matter. My point is that this idea that grey hair equates to invisibility, to over-the-hill-ness, is entirely bogus.

I write this as someone whose dark curly hair always used to be her thing. *A Room with a View* was released at the cinema when I was 13, and there was my hair, or a version of it, on the big screen. The timing was perfect. I pretty much Lucy Honeychurch-ed my way through the next two and half decades.

My dark curls were, more than anything else about my appearance, what defined me. Men loved my hair, women wanted it. I was, as a result, pretty happy with it, too. When I began to see greys, I didn't think twice about starting to dye it, first so-called 'low lights', then eventually a 'full head'. It was what all my friends and colleagues did, though I had to start a few years before those who were my age. Otherwise it was business as usual. Room. View.

Then I went grey. And even – especially? – a lifetime of hair-thing-ness didn't prepare me for the shift that followed. As I started to grow out my roots, painfully slow centimetre by centimetre, my hair became not so much my thing, as a whole other thing, a separate entity, one that merited comment and discussion, that provoked bafflement in some ('What are you trying to prove?' asked one friend) and – to my surprise – admiration in others. ('You are so brave, I wish I could do it,' was a common response from women.)

Sometimes the bafflement and the admiration seemed to co-exist.

To have grey hair as an older woman is almost countercultural these days. Globally the hair dye industry is now worth over $7 billion. As the late Nora Ephron once famously put it, 'There is a reason why 40, 50 and 60 don't look the way they used to, and it's not because of feminism . . . It's because of hair dye.'

Which is why, perversely, grey hair can make you stand out. Or at least it can if it forms part of a bigger package that also refuses to conform to societal norms: if you dress to express yourself rather than to channel those ubiquitous – and to my mind rather bland – concepts such as 'chic' and 'elegance' that are supposed to represent how older women garb themselves; if your energy, your attitude, your physicality are those of a youthful person. The end result doesn't quite compute, in a good way, and if you don't quite compute, you get noticed.

Foregrounded with clothes and make-up that have nothing to do with ideas of how an older woman should look – and if there is one concept we need to move beyond it is what I am going to call should-ness – grey hair looks cool. It signals that you are at ease with who you are; that you are authentic; that – at a deeper level – you are unafraid, be it of ageing or of anything else. I think that is why, once you have done it, and done it well, people respond so strongly, especially young people. It offers up a different road map for growing older. To confound expectations of what ageing means – and going grey in a way that looks the opposite of fusty is one way to do this – can get you seen like never before.

I actually now wish I had cut my dyed hair off all at once, gone from long to short. I think it would have been more fun to enact the change dramatically rather than to eke it out month by month. That's what an acquaintance did, and I still remember encountering the new grey-haired pixie-cropped her at a party and thinking how disencumbered she looked, how fresh. I would definitely have grown it back to its original length afterwards, but if you are in the process of growing your hair out anyway, why not embrace it fully? If you are shape-shifting – and that is what going

grey is, a step through a door from one you to another –
why not properly turn matters on their head for a
while? And why not get the process done and dusted
tout d'un coup?

Of course that's easy for me to say today. I
understand that it demands another level of bravery to
cut all your hair off. Luckily, if you don't want to go
that route, there are plenty of other things that can
make the growing-out process less painful. I would
certainly recommend embracing the shortest version
of your current style that you can manage. In the
earliest stages, Color Wow Root Cover Up can work
wonders. In the medium term you might want to have
streaks put in that balance out the colour you are now
with the colour you are becoming. A good colourist
can help make the process less painful, though don't
necessarily expect them to be keen on the idea from the
off! They make their money from the ubiquity of dyed
hair, after all.

'Clients ask me all the time, "Am I ready? Will you
tell me when I should?"' Jo Cockle, a colourist at the
John Frieda salon in London, tells me. 'Anything is

possible, but it will be a commitment initially.' She advocates patience, and expert help. If you are starting to go grey, and pondering your options, she advises 'blending your white with both lightness and shade'. This buys you some time and, should you decide eventually to go the grey route, circumvents the issue of solid regrowth lines.

Ready to enact the shift once and for all? 'I recommend adding creamy blonde sections to a whitening base, which can then be toned with shades ranging from pale silvery violets through to darker aluminium and steely tones.' Cockle also rates a colour rinse such as Redken Shades HQ and Wella's Perfecton to unify your look.

Another font of going-grey wisdom is the Instagram account @jackmartincolorist, which is full of before, during and after pictures, and lots of useful suggestions. People travel to Martin in California from all over the world, and a transformation normally takes eight hours on average in his chair. His tips include matching the natural pattern of your regrowth in order to blend the hair colour while at the same time 'adding extra wider silver strands to make the hair more glamorous'.

Changing your colour can feel dramatic at first, even frightening, but that feeling rarely lasts. When I first used to catch some odd light-coloured bit of wispiness out of the corner of my eye, I would think 'What's that?' Then I would realise that this alien thing was in fact my new hair; no, not my 'new' hair, my hair. Now, years later, my greyness is so intrinsically me that I am actually surprised when I see its original colour in an old photograph. That dark brunette just doesn't quite look like me any more. What shocks me almost as much is that my hair as it is now appears far more distinctive than it did when it was in its supposed prime. It's that visibility thing again.

There was something else that surprised me in my earliest years of being grey, but which I have grown used to now. I started to receive compliments on my skin, too. I didn't connect the two at first. I had changed nothing about my beauty regimen. Eventually I worked out what was going on. My natural hair colour was far more flattering to my skin than anything that even one of the best colourists in London had managed to pull off synthetically. As Linda Rodin, the 70-something American stylist, one of my key grey-spirations, observes, 'I sometimes think as a woman ages, dark hair is too harsh and the grey is softer and looks more harmonious.'

I believe it is easier to keep dyeing your hair if you are naturally blonde than if you are naturally brunette. The tonal difference between blonde and grey is not as large as that between brunette and grey, which means it can be less tricky, as you age, and lose pigmentation in your skin, to bridge the gap between your synthetic hair and your natural complexion. And that's before we factor in the tyranny of what, in my case, became a fortnightly visit to the hairdresser's to eradicate the line of grown-out roots that was already clearly visible; much worse if you are dark.

When I now see photographs of me taken in the later years of my hair dyeing, it surprises me how bad I looked. As Susie Orbach once said to me, 'We don't look any younger. We just look as if we dye our hair.'

That was certainly the case for me. It's another example of what she calls 'the lack of differentiation between young and old, which used to be signified by a lot of things, including grey hair'.

Indeed, the current unnatural state of affairs – 'old' women with 'young' hair – has become so normalised, certainly in the urban, professional world I inhabit, that none of us quite knows what we are looking at any more. When you sit in a hair salon full of blonde and brunette grandmothers, as I did last week, and look, really look . . . well, it's kind of odd. These women don't look young. Their hair and their faces don't match, and sometimes you can't help wondering if the face actually appears older as a result. How they look, more than anything, is how we expect them to look. They have conformed to the norms of femininity circa 2023. But no one thinks they are 25. They look like women with their grandchildren's hair.

I completely understand why women dye their hair, not least because I did it myself for years. And I don't judge anyone who continues to do so. Indeed, if you want to keep dyeing your hair, I will be giving some advice on how to make it look its best in a minute. But, whatever your personal choice, and a choice is what it should feel like, it's still worth examining what is at heart yet another manifestation of this commonplace that young is good and old is bad.

'Even if in the abstract, we think we look all right with grey hair,' says Rose Weitz, author of *Rapunzel's Daughters: What Women's Hair Tells Us About Women's Lives* (2005), 'we nonetheless feel we are losing our "real selves" if we no longer have our "real hair colour".'

As Orbach notes, 'Women think, "Will I be ignored, written off, not seen?"' She made her name with her book *Fat Is a Feminist Issue* (1978). Does that mean hair is a feminist issue too?

The fairy tale of Rapunzel is just one of the many narratives to be found across the world that equate hair to power and/or sexuality. Similarly widely known is the Biblical tale of Samson and Delilah, in which the legendary strongman loses his potency after his hair is secretly cut. In ancient Japan, aristocratic women were expected to grow their hair as long as possible and pile it in elaborately heavy styles on top of their head. This would place pressure on the brain, so the thesis went, and stop them thinking too much. In 17th-century England people would make 'witch bottles', putting some of their hair into a bottle and burying it to protect themselves from witchcraft. The stories we tell ourselves about hair today are just as potent. We dye our hair in the false belief that it will somehow ward off ageing.

Yet, of course, it can't. When the American journalist Anne Kreamer was researching her book *Going Gray: How to Embrace Your Authentic Self with Grace and Style* (2007), she sent out to hundreds of people via a survey company a set of pictures of herself and a handful of friends she had co-opted to help her. Some of the photos were of people in their thirties, some in their forties, some in their fifties. Some had naturally brown hair, some dyed it, one was grey. In each set of pictures that were sent out some of the individuals appeared as their hair actually was, and some had had their hair manipulated so that it looked grey when it wasn't, or vice versa. Everyone appeared only once in each set.

The respondents were asked to guess everyone's ages. What became clear is that hair colour made little difference to that guess. Kreamer was estimated to be 45 with brown hair, 47 with grey. Another question asked whether the respondent would 'fix this person up with a friend'. For four out of the six women who took part, 'There was a modest but consistent *advantage* [Kreamer's italics] in fix-up-ability for the gray-haired versions.'

Kreamer then tried online dating on two separate occasions, putting up a picture of herself with grey hair for three weeks, and later, after a three-month hiatus, with brown. She was surprised to receive considerably more attention when her barnet was undyed. Who are we kidding when we colour our hair? Only, perhaps, ourselves.

It's interesting too to look at what a recent phenomenon this is. Although humans have been dyeing their hair since ancient Egyptian times, it has only gone mainstream in the last few decades. This is partly because it used to be such a tricky – not to mention often disgusting – business. Pliny the Elder, writing in the first century AD, suggested that anyone who wanted black hair should let leeches putrefy for 40 days in red wine held in a leaden vessel, before then applying the unimaginably horrific results to their head.

To dye your hair tended to be considered as at best vain, at worst morally dubious. During the Roman Empire, prostitutes were required to have yellow hair to indicate their profession. In *Gone with the Wind*, first published in 1936, the prostitute Belle Watling is referred to as 'a dyed haired woman'.

Until surprisingly recently the process remained technically challenging, if not dangerous. Even in the first decades of the 20th century, if you were one of the few women who did dye their hair, you certainly didn't advertise the fact, hence those curtains at the salon. To seek to appear younger than you were, in particular, was thought to be narcissistic, not to mention delusional.

A series of technical advances, and the appearance in 1931 of Jean Harlow in the film *Platinum Blonde*, changed everything, with enthused fans dyeing their hair to match Harlow's, and billionaire producer Howard Hughes offering up a $10,000 prize to any hairdresser who could copy her shade. Ironically, the actress herself never admitted to dyeing her hair.

As of 1950, bleach was no longer required to make your hair lighter, thus reducing the damage involved. The launch of Miss Clairol Hair Color Bath – and, oh, the significance of that 'Miss' – allowed women to colour their hair at home. It was hugely successful, not only because it increased affordability but also because discretion was still paramount. Hence that slogan: 'Does she or doesn't she?'

Suddenly nice girls did (or didn't they?), and it was the lazy, letting-themselves-go ones who didn't, a different kind of loose woman. Changing your hair colour was no longer about the dark arts, about subterfuge, but about valuing yourself, revealing a better you. 'Because you're worth it' was L'Oréal's mantra.

Kreamer argues that such advertising transformed what began as 'a Hear Me Roar moment of female reinvention, of being in the world, being in control of your image, into a position of weakness – of "oh no, I've got mousy hair, I'm not attractive." '

The last century has seen the entry of women *en masse* into the workplace, and along with it the perceived need to look as young as possible in a competitive market. Then there has been the concomitant transformation in our romantic lives, in which sex and being sexy aren't just for young people, and in which you can end up back on the market at any age and, again, feel the need to look as young as possible to compete. Women didn't used to want to look young, particularly. They wanted to look the best possible version of their age. Now many of us would love to be mistaken for our daughters, and there is no more one-stop way to kid ourselves that this might happen than to erase our greys. It is out with ageing gracefully; ideally, out with ageing at all.

It's one of the strangest dichotomies of our era. We have more freedom than we have had for millennia. We have the capacity to self-determine who we are, how we live and – relatedly – how we look, like never before. And we have turned this into a new kind of prison – 'we' meaning society as a whole, but also we women in particular. That's hardly surprising. We have been trained for (again) millennia to internalise other people's expectations, whether it is the colour our hair is supposed to be, or the size of our thighs, or the degree to which we are (or, as is more often the case, aren't) outspoken.

As the American essayist Jia Tolentino writes in *Trick Mirror: Reflections on Self-Delusion* (2019), 'The ideal woman has always been generic. I bet you can picture the version of her that runs the show today. She's of indeterminate age, but resolutely youthful . . . She looks like an Instagram [post] – which is to say, an ordinary woman reproducing the lessons of the marketplace, which is how an ordinary woman evolves into the ideal. The process requires maximum obedience on the part of the woman in question, and – ideally – her genuine enthusiasm, too. This woman is sincerely interested in whatever the market demands of her (good looks, the impression of indefinitely extended youth, advanced skills in self-presentation and self-surveillance) . . . The ideal woman, in other words, is always optimising.'

Always optimising. That's certainly what dyeing my hair was a version of for me. But I began to feel tyrannised by the dyeing schedule, its regularity and the related expense. I was also starting to think more about how to reduce the 'toxic load' in my life – eating organically, switching beauty and household products – and it seemed ridiculous still to be whacking chemicals on my head over a dozen times a year. (Dark hair dye is considered the most toxic. A couple of friends had to stop dyeing their hair when their face began to swell up. Google 'para-phenylenediamine' if you want to scare yourself into going grey.)

And also for me, I came to realise, hair *was* a feminist issue. I was getting annoyed about the whole fandango. Did I really have to pretend my hair was something other than what it was to look my best, to feel attractive, when men didn't do the same?

One of my happiest discoveries of recent years is that I didn't. Even my most avid nay-sayers loved my new look. A couple of them started growing out their own greys. I experienced something similar more recently when, having been advised by almost everyone *not* to have a fringe, it's now the subject of much admiration. 'You will regret it if you don't like it,' said one well-meaning friend. *Au contraire.* I would have regretted it if I hadn't tried it. What's the worst that could happen? You grow your fringe out. You dye your hair back. The alternative? A missed opportunity has been well and truly missed.

What I now hear a lot from other women about my grey is that it is all right for me because I have the 'right hair' or the 'right skin tone'. Yes, I have gone a 'good grey', but they wouldn't if they tried to do the same. The theory I have been told over and again is that if you were originally a brunette and, even better, like me, a dark one, you can go grey, but that it won't work well for anyone else.

Initially I didn't have a riposte to that. I could only take them at their word. Since then, however, I have been collecting fellow greyers, women I have met or who have contacted me, many of whom had a starting point, be it in terms of hair colour and/or texture, skin tone or all three, that was entirely different from my own. I now know that anyone can go a good grey.

What's important is that you keep your overall look youthful. We discussed skincare and make-up in the last chapter. We will talk about staying physically in shape in the next – good posture and mobility are two of the most potent beauty tools we have – and about making the right fashion choices in the one after that. Part of it, too, is having the right haircut: something that is contemporary; that isn't try-hard, but that is now rather than then. Denise Boomkens, who is currently struggling with hair loss, tells me, 'It's a bit of a challenge, but you can do a lot by keeping your hair healthy and modern-looking.'

It is certainly important that you maintain your hair in the best condition possible. Dryness can be one of the biggest issues we face as we get older. 'Hair that has always appeared glossy and sleek can suddenly seem bushy and matt,' says Jo Cockle. And that's whether you stop dyeing it or continue to colour it. The texture of grey hair is just different. I now do a five-minute hair mask every time I wash my hair. My favourite is Living Proof's Anti-Frizz Intense Moisture Mask. If you don't have issues with frizz, then that same brand's Perfect Hair Day Weightless Mask is the best option.

I love Living Proof generally. All of its products are free of silicons, parabens and phthalates, and haven't been tested on animals. All of them – or at least all of them I have now tried, which is a fair few – deliver on what they say on the tin. One illustration of note is that Living Proof eschews the silicon used by many other hair brands, because – who knew? – it turns out that silicon is as good at attracting dirt to the hair as it is at smoothing it. A lose-win if ever there was one.

I used to find that my greys had a tendency to yellow, which can be caused by chemical residues both in hair products and in the water itself. I used to use a shampoo and conditioner with a blue or purple tint occasionally, even though I wasn't delighted by the chemicals this entailed. Since switching to Living Proof and fitting a water filter in my shower, I haven't had any issues.

I also wrap my hair in a 90cm² silk kerchief at night when I want to keep it looking smooth for as long as possible. I fold the square once to make a triangle, put the long folded edge at the nape of my neck and, catching the hair within the silk, tie the two corners in a knot at the top of my hairline. I then tuck the loose edges up and under the tied circle to create something akin to an impromptu bonnet. Silke London produces ready-made options as an alternative.

All in all, I haven't faded to grey. Quite the opposite.

But the route I have taken isn't the only one, of course. Should you choose to continue to dye, Cockle warns against 'solid permanent shades. The way to go is to introduce super-fine baby-lights in varying depths and tones.' If you are struggling, as I used to, with regrowth that seems to kick in the second you leave the salon, she also recommends 'wearing a lighter shade around the hairline' in order to minimise that telltale dark line.

If your original hair colour is dark, you will probably need to go lighter in order to chime with your changing skin tone. (The number of pigment-containing cells in your epidermis decreases as you age.) There's a reason why Anna Wintour tweaked that signature brunette bob of hers to be something more akin to blonde. Fading to blonde is just fine, too.

7

Your Body Beautiful

If I asked you to tell me everything you liked about your body, what would you have to say? How long would the list be? And if I asked you what you didn't? I'd wager that list would be longer. Women are bombarded with ideas of what their bodies should and shouldn't be like from a young age.

Should? Shouldn't? We have already discussed how these are the world's least helpful words. But they are difficult to escape, especially for women, programmed until very recently to exist primarily for others, to be seen more than heard and, resultantly, to police themselves into conformity.

No wonder we often end up viewing our bodies in a

way that's akin to those old-fashioned diagrams of a cow that you used to find in butcher's shops, each bit of us marked off and considered in isolation (the sirloin, the flank), some bits too small, other bits too large, very little of us exactly right.

It was the fashion designer Carolina Herrera who once told me that the most important thing every woman should have in her wardrobe was – wait for it! – a full-length mirror. She is right: it's a great way to get to understand properly what suits you and why. I also think a long mirror is a valuable tool for starting to rewire your attitude to your body.

Stand in front of that mirror naked every morning for a week or two and appraise your body as a whole. Don't immediately start analysing the bits of it that you don't like. In fact, you are not allowed to say to yourself that you don't like anything. Take it all in, in one piece. Admire it in all its wonderment. And give thanks. Every body, whatever its shape or size, is a miraculous thing, the ship on which we sail through the waters of life.

Any woman I have ever asked about her physicality has always – in however fantastic shape someone else might deem her to be – reeled off a catalogue of dissatisfactions. I am no exception. Or at least I wasn't. I wanted my hips to be narrower, my thighs to be thinner, my boobs to be bouncier . . . I mean, really, how long have you got? Not long enough, probably. I will spare you.

Next, look in your mirror, find one thing in particular that you want to give thanks for and give a reason why. And so much the better if this reason is related to function rather than form, to what this part of your body does for you rather than how it looks. If you can find a different thing each day for a week or so then so much the better. If it can be something that you usually berate yourself for then that's better still.

When I do this exercise these days – it's worth checking in with it every so often *ad infinitum* – I often choose to focus on my supposedly big thighs and give thanks for how strong they make me; how they are part of what makes me able to out-walk almost anyone. As for those aforementioned frown lines between my eyes, I give thanks for the visual reminder they are giving me to stress less; to be in the present rather than to exist in my head.

When it comes to my most notable physical stigmata, a large scar on my abdomen from childhood surgery that I have spent a lifetime doing my best not to see nor think about, these days I see it, truly see it, and I love it and thank it for being the means by which I was kept alive. Then there are my boobs . . . OK, so I admit that I would still like them to be bouncier, but no one's perfect, right?! I am who I am, boobs and all.

We are brought up to believe that our bodies are us, but not in an accepting way, not in a way that makes us grateful for having a physical form that serves us day in, day out, year after year. Instead we inherit the notion that if our particular body isn't good enough – whatever 'good enough' happens to mean – then neither are we. The result is that many of us also end up feeling that our bodies *aren't* us; that our physicality imprisons us or holds us to ransom because it doesn't conform to what we want it to be. The fact that none of this makes much sense is indicative of the confused state we are in.

And so we do what we are told to do, what we are told we should – that word again – do. We police our eating and jog or gym our way towards the dimensions that are supposed to be ours. Rare is the woman who isn't permanently running some kind of calories-in-to-calories-out counter in her head. Even the cleverest and most empowered of us can't shake off the petty monitoring, such is its hardwiring in our collective consciousness. It's just that most women aren't honest about it.

The columnist Janice Turner wrote in *The Times* in 2022 about finding her elderly mother's 'scribbled daily records: boiled egg (60), 1 slice toast (75), ½ grapefruit (42)'. Turner herself, a super-brain if ever there was one, admits that 'the involuntarily daily calculation fills my head. I can tell you foods which are calorie bargains (Jaffa Cakes, only 46 each!) or calorie traps ("luxury" granola: 4 billion per bowl). That inner ticker tape of denial v indulgence, good v bad foods, is both joyless and pointless. I don't remember my mother ever getting much thinner, just losing her self-control by teatime and miserably eating a scone.'

How many of us have lived – or continue to live – a version of that setup? I know I did for years. Either I was being good, exhaustingly sugar-free, minimal-fats good, or I was being bad, blow it all to the winds bad, eating things that I thought I wanted but, looking back, I might well have wanted a bit of, but probably didn't want half a packet of. I never had an eating disorder, but in retrospect I probably had some kind of disordered eating. I was always monitoring, even when what I was monitoring was my not-monitoring.

In her book *Bodies* (2009), Susie Orbach writes of the modern obsession with 'perfectibility' and how, in her consulting room, 'whatever their other emotional predicaments and conflicts, concern for the body is nearly always folded into them.' She talks about a modern 'crisis' around the body, about how it is no longer 'something that unfolds organically from birth . . . something essentially stable'.

In her equally seminal *The Beauty Myth* (1990), Naomi Wolf notes that it was when 'women breached the power structure' in the 1980s that 'eating disorders rose exponentially and cosmetic surgery became the fastest-growing medical specialty.'

Where did the so-called thin ideal come from? In *Unbearable Weight: Feminism, Western Culture and the*

Body (1995), Susan Bordo argues that it's about 'the tantalising ideal of a well-managed self in which all is kept in order'. That this has had a greater hold over women than men is because 'throughout dominant Western religious and philosophical traditions, the capacity for self-management is decisively coded as male. In contrast all those bodily spontaneities – hunger, sexuality, the emotions – seen as needful of containment and control have been culturally constructed . . . as female.' Well, quite.

And so, to follow Bordo's argument, modern women – or at least those in 'late modern Western societies' – have used their bodies to demonstrate to others that they can do, be, live as men do. Which feeds in, too, to a slightly more positive reading, namely that thinness symbolises 'not so much the containment of female desire, but its liberation from a domestic, reproductive destiny'.

I think Bordo is onto something. Certainly we set out to stage-manage our bodies in such a way that they will perform to the world at large an idea about us that we believe to be in our best interests. And along the way, as always happens when we think about our audience more than ourselves, we lose sight of ourselves.

That idea of 'always optimising' that Jia Tolentino wrote about is just as prevalent as ever, even though we live in a society that claims to have become better at self-acceptance. 'The psychological parasite of the ideal woman has evolved to survive in an ecosystem that pretends to resist her,' she writes. 'If a woman starts to resist an aesthetic, like an overapplication of Photoshop, the aesthetic just changes to suit us; the power of the ideal image never actually wanes.'

What I wasn't doing for all those years of 'always optimising' was checking in with what my body truly wanted. My responses to food were psychological, coming from my head and heart rather than my stomach. When I began to listen to my true appetites I learned that, yes, my body still liked Party Rings, but it probably only wanted a couple, and that it liked spinach just as much.

It was the same story when I began to listen to my body around exercise. I tended to be all or nothing in this regard, too. Either I wasn't particularly motivated, or I was caning it at the gym. I knew from my teens that I was happier when I was fit. What I didn't properly register until my forties was that when I really pushed myself at the gym I would feel great immediately afterwards but deeply depleted a couple of hours later, and that it would take me a long time properly to recover.

With a big job at the time that already depleted me, stressed in more ways than I cared to admit, the last thing I needed was to deplete and stress my body further. In the West we tend to think of exercise as perforce effortful, as another kind of output. Eastern disciplines such as t'ai chi and chi gong, in contrast, are concerned with drawing energy inwards in order to build and consolidate that aforementioned *chi*, your life force.

In his book *How to Eat, Move and Be Healthy* (2004), the American holistic health practitioner and corrective exercise specialist Paul Chek offers an approach that can bespoked to suit what your body needs for maximum health and efficacy. It is not about exercising more; indeed often – for those who are living stressful lives – it's the reverse. First you fill out his questionnaire, which asks you about everything from how often you wake up at night to whether you have any skin conditions. Your answers determine which zones of your body most need attention, from zone 1 (the pelvis, legs and feet) to zone 6 (the upper neck, face and head). The so-called zone exercises Chek then offers up don't, he promises, 'fatigue – they *energise!*' [Chek's emphasis.]

Even a walking meditation can transform your energy levels. With as much mindfulness as you can muster, the aim is 'to walk as slowly as possible,' writes Chek. 'The key is always to be moving, but moving very slowly, like a cat sneaking up on a bird, yet staying very relaxed. With slow walking you should become very much in touch with the now, the moment. The slower you go, the more *chi* flow you will create and the better your balance will become.'

What I also grew increasingly weary about with my former gym life was the degree to which so many exercise approaches seemed to be aimed at changing the aesthetics of certain bits of my body. If I was busy learning to love my thighs, how helpful was it to be given a training programme at the gym specifically designed to 'sculpt' them? Besides, by that stage in the game I had come to accept that my bodily proportions were what they were. Everything could get smaller, or everything could get bigger. This idea of micromanaging one part over another is another pup we have been sold.

The secret to finding your body beautiful – and that possessive is key, because it is yours and yours alone, calibrated to your natural appetites and needs – is to give it what it needs, which is care and attention that are wholly positive. It's not about shoulds or shouldn'ts. It's not about someone else's rules. It's about listening to your body rather than overriding it.

It's also not about ignoring your body in the other sense: being self-indulgent and/or lazy. One of the biggest age-enhancing options we have is to keep ourselves feeling as physically strong and alive as possible, not in a try-hard way, but again with that idea of effortless effortfulness. The Greek philosopher Alcmaeon noted that 'Health is harmony; disease is a disturbance of harmony.' Harmony is what we are looking for in all aspects of our lives; our age, and the wisdom it opens up to us, can help us access it far more easily than a younger person.

The Roman poet Juvenal came up two millennia ago with the idea of *mens sana in corpore sano*, a sound mind in a sound body. The idea of the bodymind as an inseparable entity has been central to Eastern therapeutic traditions for even longer, a concept that we are finally catching up with in the West. Look after your body and your mind will follow, and vice versa. Consistently eating too little is as damaging as eating too much. Consistently over-exercising is as problematic as never doing any physical activity. Eating and exercise both represent ways either to check in with the bodymind or to check out.

Certainly the psychological shift that has happened in me since I finally tuned into an approach to food and exercise that works for me has been profound. To be stronger and more flexible at 50 than I was at 20 has been one of my life's greatest surprises so far, as well as one of its greatest joys. And it's never too late. Last year, I started teaching a weekly yoga class. I love to watch my students, most of them beginners, start to find their yogic way. I love to bear witness to how their practice changes, and with it their physical capabilities. But even I am surprised sometimes by some of the feedback. 'I feel so much stronger,' one woman told me the other day. 'I think I might go on a date.' It was just another illustration of the intertwined workings of the bodymind. Feel strong in your body, feel strong enough to try dating. (And, golly, do you need to gird your loins, as I discuss in chapter 10, but it *is* worth it.) To feel strong and flexible in your body is to feel strong and flexible in the world. We are not our body, just as we are not our face. Yet, just like our face, our body can reveal deeper truths about who we are.

The late Italian yogi Vanda Scaravelli, who was famous for her remarkable backbends up to her death at 91 in 1999, only started to practise in her fifties. There are pictures of her as an old lady with her feet on the floor, her back bending so deeply that her hands are almost on the floor behind her, yet held in the air just so. She displays strength and suppleness that would be notable in someone in their twenties.

Scaravelli's book *Awakening the Spine* (1991) is not only a yoga instruction manual but a paean to the potentiality of old age done well. 'Goethe was 82 when he completed *Faust*,' she notes. 'Giuseppe Verdi wrote his sparkling comic opera *Falstaff* at a mere 79 . . . Picasso's vitality even in his nineties was proverbial.'

She believed that it was a flexible spine that was the physical key to unlocking a feeling of youthfulness, but much of what she writes has a deeper application. The focus in her book is not only on learning how to backbend, slowly growing more comfortable with a pose that demands both weight (in the lower body) and lightness (in the upper body), but on larger truths around life in general, and ageing in particular.

'We have been trained, during the first part of our lives, to struggle, to achieve,' she writes. 'Now we have to work in the opposite direction, by letting go, giving place to a different kind of action (if we can call it an action), an "un-doing action". This will stop the habitual process of doing, which has become mechanical.'

Part of that process of un-doing is also about

acceptance; about acknowledging that where you are at is where you are at; about never – *ever* – beating yourself up about *anything*. Failure isn't failure when it comes to weight or fitness or anything else. It's an opportunity to learn. It's a step on the road to success. I frequently mess up; become physically lazy; greedily eat food because my head rather than my body wants it. I just don't see it as messing up any more. I see it as being a work in progress; more than that, of being alive.

Here's another example of a late adopter. At 70 – six years ago as I write this – Joan MacDonald, a Canadian retiree, was obese, on medication for high blood pressure among other things, and suffering from painful arthritis. With the help of her daughter, a personal trainer whose expertise is weightlifting, MacDonald has transformed the way she looks and feels. She is now 70lb lighter than when she started out, with – much more importantly – a huge shift in her physical functionality and all her health markers.

As MacDonald wrote on her Instagram account @trainwithjoan, 'I never thought I would be "here". I didn't even know that "here" existed. I just thought

I would be a slightly less fat version of what I started out as, and hopefully off my medications . . . But here I am now, grateful that I never gave up . . . Wherever you are, do not give up!'

Weightlifting isn't my thing, but it has become MacDonald's, and that is all that matters. Yoga *is* my thing, but it may not be yours. Again, that doesn't matter. All that matters is for you to find your way to a form of movement that suits you mentally and physically, so much so that you want to do it almost every day for the rest of your life.

We are designed to move. Maintaining that mobility becomes more important than ever as you get older. To keep your joints as oiled as possible is to avoid that tendency towards ever-so-slightly-jerky, tin-man-style walking that many people develop as they stiffen up over the decades. To walk youthfully is to appear youthful.

It is common in yoga to hear parallels drawn between physical and mental flexibility: that body-mind connection once again. But other physical practitioners talk about it too. In *Stretching Scientifically: A Guide to Flexibility Training* (1988), Thomas Kurz writes,

'Mental rigidity – the inability to abandon fixed ideas while solving problems – is usually accompanied by a low level of physical flexibility, perhaps due to the connection between flexibility and coordination.'

Load-bearing exercise is also essential. Wolff's law – a medical concept developed in the 19th century by German anatomist and surgeon Julius Wolff – shows that bone will remodel itself in response to loading, which in turn stimulates a process known as mechano-transduction. This increases the electrochemical feedback that enables the rest of your body to know what your bones need in order to stay healthy. To maintain your skeleton is to maintain your posture; to stand straight is the ultimate one-stop way to appear immediately more youthful.

The body is, among other things, a storage system. It holds emotions and experiences. Unless you don't let it. The more toxic those emotions and experiences, the worse it is, as Dr Bessel van der Kolk explores in his seminal work on trauma, the tellingly entitled *The Body Keeps the Score: Brain, Mind, and Body in the Healing of Trauma* (2014). Shaking things up, literally, can be hugely helpful in moving anything that's stuck. (I have already mentioned the *chi* machine, and gently shaking everything you are holding in your body is just what it does.) There's a reason why traditionally in much of the world the mourning process has included some sort of dancing. And that's another reason why you need to keep moving.

What I would advocate is finding a physical activity – or indeed activities – that gives you a narrative progression; that is focused on function rather than on form, on becoming more skilled at something; that requires you to engage your brain as well as your body. That's one of the many aspects of yoga that I love. It is not about striving – probably unsuccessfully – to make your tummy flatter and your bottom rounder. (I mean, honestly, the contradictory nonsense of this stuff.) It's about working at what your body can do. It's about discovering new physical pathways, which in turn create new neural pathways.

It's also about having fun in the process. Doing anything under sufferance impacts your body differently from if you do it with joy, and that includes exercise. We need to be playful. Carrie Owerko is an American yogi who, at 59, has the strength and flexibility of someone decades younger. 'As we age, play – and learning new things – becomes even more essential for brain and body health and overall well-being,' she says. Here's to play. Always.

It is so exciting to me that every year, if I just show up on my mat regularly, new capabilities open up to me. With Vanda Scaravelli as my blueprint, I hope that will be the case into my nineties. I can't do a backbend anywhere near as deep as hers yet. I am only just getting started on this aspect of my practice really. But I aim to pull off Scaravelli levels of bendiness by the time other people my age are using a zimmer frame.

I have also thus far kept cellulite entirely at bay courtesy of a combination of practices designed to supercharge my lymphatic system. These include dry body brushing (my favourite brushes come from Hydrea), body drumming (another brilliant gadget from Hayo'u Method) and hot-cold-hot showers (they really aren't so bad if you end on hot). Then there's my obsession with getting upside down as much as possible, which is also great for increasing circulation. If the idea of learning headstand – never mind handstand – makes you blanch, I can highly recommend a gadget called a FeetUp® Trainer, which allows even someone inexperienced to invert safely.

There is a weight and shape that your body is supposed to be, at which you feel happy, strong and alive, and only you can find your way there. However, there are a few approaches and a few people who will help you on your way. It may be that you are already there. In which case, congratulations. You have managed on your own to achieve that balance which should be simple but which society makes it very hard for most of us to find. If this is you, you will probably be used to checking in with what really serves you in terms of what you eat and how you exercise, but it still won't hurt to pick up some more tips. For everyone else, prepare yourself for a profound transformation of how you feel about your body and, very possibly, by extension, of your body itself.

There are two books that were a complete game-changer for me with food, both with titles that I would have once found difficult to – no pun intended – swallow. The first is *Women, Food and God: An Unexpected Path to Almost Everything* (2010) by Geneen Roth, who suffered from bulimia when she was young. The second is the aforementioned *Within: A Spiritual Awakening to Love & Weight Loss* by Dr Habib Sadeghi.

You may already be baulking at the titles. How can your weight have anything to do with spirituality, you may be thinking. I would urge you to read one or both anyway. In the meantime, here are a few of the best insights from both.

Roth, who struggled with compulsive eating for decades and now runs retreats designed to help women liberate themselves from an antipathetic relationship with food, believes 'our relationship with food is an exact microcosm of our relationship with life itself. I believe we are walking, talking expressions of our deepest convictions; everything we believe about love, fear, transformation and God is revealed in how, when and what we eat . . . God – however we define him or her – is on our plates.'

Roth believes that we use eating – or indeed not

eating – to escape aspects of ourselves or our lives with which we are uncomfortable. 'Women turn to food when they are not hungry because they are hungry for something they can't name: a connection to what is beyond the concerns of daily life.' Sadeghi writes similarly: 'In regard to weight loss, I say that 90% of success comes from what you put in your heart/mind, and that diet and exercise only count for about 10%.'

We confuse a spiritual – in the broadest sense of the word – hunger, an awareness that something is missing in ourselves and/or our world, with physical hunger. Food becomes a proxy, and we use it not to nurture ourselves but as a distraction from ourselves, or as a means to reward or punish ourselves, the former – when it comes to overeaters – in truth a kind of punishment in disguise.

For two decades Roth transmuted 'the suffering I felt about anything – my parents' marriage, my boyfriend's . . . death, my chubby moon face – . . . in my relationship with food. Overeating was my way to punish and shame myself; each time I gained weight, each time I failed at a diet, I proved to myself that my deepest fear was true: I was pathetic and doomed and didn't deserve to live.'

My own story is less boldface. Yet I can see now that I was always trying to perfect myself and my body through what I did or didn't eat, rather than nourishing myself, or that I had fallen off the wagon and was eating more rubbish than – if I could have just tuned into myself – I actually wanted. My body was something else – like my job, my relationship, my place in the world – that was to be strived for; that I couldn't allow just to be. I was rollercoastering rather than following my path.

How to find your way out of this mess? By using your bodily wisdom. By removing the psychodrama with which our society imbues the act of eating, with everything designated as either good or bad. Forget being good or bad. Just be you. Nothing is disallowed. All that is disallowed is eating when you are not hungry.

I have found that intermittent fasting works brilliantly for me in this regard, helping me to eat according not to some arbitrary timetable, but to my body's particular needs. If I listen to my body, it doesn't really want breakfast (which was, in fact, a concept only cooked up in the 19th century, and which became dominant largely due to assiduous commercialisation by Kellogg's). It took a while for me to recalibrate – habit is a powerful thing – but I can now happily wait until 2pm to eat, which makes it easy for me to adhere to a so-called 16–8 fasting window, limiting my food and calorific drink intake to a set period of eight hours per day. I am actually hungrier for lunch earlier on the rare occasions when I do eat on rising, a common phenomenon explained by the fact that the act of eating releases ghrelin, the so-called hunger hormone.

Whether fasting is for you or not, learn to check in with the difference between what is known as 'mouth hunger' and true 'stomach hunger'. By all means have some chocolate. But eat it slowly, eat it mindfully, really taste it, and stop the second you feel satiated.

Yes, mindfulness. That word again. Your body knows when it's properly hungry and for what, and when you have eaten enough for it not to be. As with all those other aspects of our lives, we are given other people's maps – be it our parents telling us to clear our plate, or the latest diet telling us what (not) to eat – when in truth our own innate cartography is the only one that counts.

Think about it. Have you ever forced yourself past your natural satiation point because something is so delicious, or because you are out with friends, or going through a devil-may-care phase? I know I have. Have you ever eaten because you were tired, bored or unhappy? Guilty as charged. And, conversely, have you ever denied yourself food when you were hungry, or made yourself eat something you don't really like because it was 'healthy'?

Roth gives the women who come to her retreats daily eating exercises in which they receive a small cup with three different foodstuffs in it, perhaps a grape, a tortilla chip and a piece of chocolate. You have to look at each item before you eat it, hold it up and really look at it, and then you have to eat it slowly, preciously, with your full attention, properly tasting it on your tongue. You have to check in with how it makes you feel, and also how having so little of it makes you feel.

'You have to be willing to go all the way,' says Roth. 'To understand that food is a stand-in for love and possibility.' As Sadeghi puts it, 'Your heart and body have their own language, and in order to speak it, we need to bypass that "thinking" watcher-at-the-gate: your brain.'

There is something else going on, too. In his Chinese Medicine-based book *Recipes for Self-Healing* (1999), the British nutritionist Daverick Leggett argues that it is not only about what you eat, but about *how* you eat. You need to eat slowly and calmly, so that your digestive system can work at its best. Your attitude to what you are eating will also have an impact.

'To be nourished by food, both mind and body need to be open to receiving its nourishment,' Leggett writes. 'Eating the "perfect" diet is no guarantee of being fully nourished . . . Two people can eat the same meal but receive it differently. One person sitting happily with a cream tea, clear in the belief that "a little of what you fancy does you good", is predisposed to digest it well and be nourished. Another person sitting with the belief that a cream tea is fattening, bad for the arteries and an indulgence, is predisposed to digest it badly.'

Factoring in other Eastern principles such as not eating too much raw food (lightly cooked vegetables are much easier to digest, for example) and not eating raw food in the evening (when it is likely to sit undigested in the stomach overnight and ferment) can also have a dramatic impact on how you digest, which in turn can shape how you feel. The stomach is called the second brain for a reason. Part of our nervous system – the so-called enteric nervous system – extends along our entire digestive tract. Just one of the other fallacies we have also been told: that you can never eat too much salad.

It's really difficult when you start to consume differently, because most of us are so hardwired to finish our plate, or worry about what is or isn't on it, or not to allow ourselves an actual plate in the first place. But if you keep on showing up to the practice – because it is a practice – eventually it starts to become almost discombobulatingly simple. You eat just what you want, calmly and slowly, in exactly the amount you want, when you are hungry. You stop when you have had enough. It's a way of life, not a diet. It's you doing you, and as a result becoming you.

I have also found my own digestion – always sluggish – to be transformed by taking a probiotic, and above all by a product called Oxytech, a so-called colon conditioner from Dulwich Health. This has addressed an array of long-term issues encompassing constipation, irritable bowel and candida. According to Dulwich Health's website, Oxytech delivers ozone (O_3) and oxygen (O_2) into the colon, which then breaks debris into pieces so that it can be easily and gently eliminated. Unlike laxatives, it has no negative impact on natural peristalsis, so long-term use isn't a problem. It is not an overstatement to say it has changed my life.

Sadeghi notes that 'when we eat consciously, we are satiated sooner and consume less, because it's the sensation of the food that satisfies us – not the quantity.' Certainly Roth reports that many of the women who go on her retreats end up becoming the slimmest they have been in their lives. They break out of the cycle of binge and purge, and find their way to whatever size it was they were supposed to be all along. They end up practising moderation, because moderation is what the body craves. They come to realise, after years of 'eating to resist and rebel and fight', as Roth puts it, 'that eating can finally be – and always was – for you and only you.'

8

Making Fashion Your Friend

I am a fashion journalist. Of course I think clothes matter, and I always have. Yet I have come to feel this more strongly than ever in the last few years. At 30 I certainly understood that clothes could be a route to self-expression, not to mention fun. I had also already learned from experience that clothes could empower and augment me; that the right coral silk jacket, by way of one long-disintegrated example that I still hold close to my heart, could provide a kind of existential armour in, say, a work meeting where I was the only woman, and at least a decade younger than everyone else.

What's more, I understood that you could deploy your clothing choices either to conform or not to conform; to belong to a group or set yourself apart from it. Take that coral jacket again. None of my male colleagues would have been able to get away with wearing anything that colourful. (More on this later.) Dressing in a way that underlined my difference in the group, rather than dressing to fit in, while still adhering to certain rules around what looked professional, was a statement of self-belief, of confidence, and I know it was read as such by others.

Indeed, when I was eventually promoted, the woman who took over my job asked me if we could go for lunch so she could solicit my advice. To my surprise she didn't only want to talk about the nature of the job itself. She also wanted to ask me where to buy good colourful jackets, not to mention bright lipsticks, another variety of armoury for me.

Even so, it was only much more recently that I realised the degree to which you can use clothes to challenge other people's idea about what group you belong to and/or what the true nature of that group is. What you wear can help you to defy a categorisation that doesn't serve you.

I didn't need to use clothes in this way until I grew older. That was when I found that my experience of who I was becoming – and in particular the fact that I found getting older made me feel more, not less; expanded, not shrunk – was at odds with how others thought an older woman should feel.

I came to understand that my idea of 50 – as the most fully realised, not to mention joyful point I have been in my life so far – is not in line with our society's ideas of 50. And while I know that the most important ways I challenge those misconceptions around age are how I am in my head (my thoughts) and how I am in the world (my actions), I also know that how I present myself can signal my divergence from clichéd ideas about ageing as a move into irrelevance, if not obsolescence.

How I dress has a huge impact on what kind of 50-year-old the world takes me to be. Whether we like it or not, people make decisions about us within seconds. First impressions – not to mention second and third ones – count. And our clothes are a key element in those impressions. That's why making choices about what you wear isn't mere whimsy, but a way to make manifest who you really are. Fashion that feels true to and expressive of your inner self, not fly-by-night or inauthentic, is a way not only to be seen but to also to be heard. That we older women should render ourselves visible in order also to help render ourselves audible is, in a society that doesn't want us to be either, incredibly important. This is not just a personal act; it's a political one. And it's forging a new path, providing fresh inspiration, for those women who will follow in our footsteps.

When I show up in a sharp black trouser suit worn with a purple Snoopy T-shirt and lilac furry shoes, for example – one of my default current ensembles – no one is going to mistake me for fusty, boring, conventional, over-the-hill or any of those other words that the unwise might confuse with growing older. At the same time my suit communicates adulthood, competency and – when I wear it in a work-related context – professionalism.

I am a slightly confusing proposition, and not easily categorised as a result. People have to give me the benefit of their full attention in order to attempt to work me out, and once I have got that attention, I have the time and the space to show them who I really am.

It only takes one slightly unexpected piece, one off-kilter element, to transform a look from predictable to box-fresh, like when I offset a pretty white broderie blouse, simple jeans and trainers with a sequin-embellished combat jacket from Essentiel Antwerp, one of my favourite brands for an adult-appropriate flourish. I get at least one compliment on that jacket every time I wear it, and it's usually from a woman or a man who looks to be a couple of decades younger than me. My clothes – combined with my grey hair and my statement lipstick – get me seen. This then opens the door to me being heard.

Certainly you can go head-to-toe unconventional, but it's less intimidating when you start to change things up simply to add in a quirky pair of shoes, or some interesting jewellery, or a jacket that gets people talking, and leave the rest well alone.

That's one of the things I remember most clearly about when I first started going to the catwalk shows. The most powerful women in the audience were then decades older than me. Some of them were very 'fashion', very full-throttle. Many of them, however, were far more classically dressed, but there was nearly always something unusual in the mix.

I recall seeing one woman, a vision in camel, who had a pair of glasses with frames that I, a fraction her age, would never have dared to wear. She looked fantastic. I remember another individual, in white and black, who was sporting a mad pair of shoes. She too looked, yes, you guessed it, fantastic.

The ultimate example has always been the designer Miuccia Prada, 73, who might offset vintage diamonds and aquamarines plus a plain white shirt with – as was the case when I interviewed her once – a skirt made of large wooden beads that made me think of those car-seat covers designed to give you an impromptu back massage.

There is no one more aware of the contradictions of fashion than Mrs Prada, as she is known at her brand headquarters in Milan. She once told me, an ironic smile twinkling on her face, that she worries that 'everyone who is smart says they hate fashion.' It is 'so easy for men to look right,' she continued, and so much more complicated – given all the choices they face – for women.

She proceeded to tell me of her own love of wearing 'men's heavy shoes, skirt, shirt, V-necked sweater. In Italy we call it *racchia*, which means boring. Boring bad.' Another smile. 'Aaaah. I love it. You know, like a nun. It makes you feel so relaxed. I guess it is what it is like for a man. It is like giving up on the problem.'

At the same time she described herself as saddened by her girlfriends who have given up on fashion; who, as she put it, 'hide because they don't want to express themselves through clothes, who reject the feminine point of view.' For her, clothes are an extension of her mind, so much so that she has a tendency not even to check herself in the mirror. 'I should start! But I know that what I have in my mind is stronger than looking right in my clothes.'

Whenever you see Miuccia Prada there is always something about her ensemble that is unusual or interesting; there is always something that makes you want to hear what she has to say, what she is thinking.

For me it's about short-circuiting people's expectations, maybe not a whole lot, but a little. We have spoken already about map-making; about how it behoves us to keep on making new ones. We have also spoken about how most people give up or, at the very least, dial their inner cartographer down at some point. To live dynamically and expansively is not only about you redrawing your own maps but also about nudging other people into redrawing their maps that relate to you. Clothes are a great way to stop them falling back on old assumptions and make them take a fresh look at you as an individual rather than some kind of prototype.

That is why I have become more aesthetically outspoken than I was when I was younger. Why I have become more embracing of colour, pattern and what might be called a certain eccentricity. Why I dress to please myself more than I ever have in my life. Just as I now worry less about what people think of me in all aspects of my life, just as I have become better at living my truth, so I have become better at dressing my truth.

I am with Denise Boomkens when she says, 'I am not interested in looking sexy, or classy. It's about dressing beyond the rules.'

This isn't about going crazy. It's not about dressing as if you are in panto – unless you want it to be, of course. Much as I salute the personal style of many of the women on the Instagram feed @advancedstyle, for example, and recommend it as an exemplification of how not to age quietly and invisibly, I myself don't want to look too theatrical. It's not for me, the big hats, retro styling and head-to-toe bonkersness approach, but I admire those women for whom it is. I, in contrast, always want to look current, relevant, contemporary, which means lightly referencing trends while still embracing the things I have always loved and that have always loved me. For me Boomkens' @andbloom feed is an unbeatable resource when it comes to ideas for ageing stylishly.

Of course, you may already know exactly how to dress your best. You may not need any help from me. But if you do need to find your way to your personal style, a great way to start is with a word. Yes, just a word.

Imagine yourself at a party. Someone who doesn't know you glimpses you across a crowded room. What is the one word you want to come into their head when they see you? It may be that a word comes to mind immediately. It may not. Don't panic if so. Sit with it a while and see what eventually arises. I have known this to take a couple of days for some people. What I will say is that the longer it takes, the more this would suggest that you haven't got a clear idea of how you dress and whether it serves you. That's hardly surprising. We aren't taught this stuff. We are all just making it up as we go along, usually guided by elements of our subconscious – those maps again – that may or may not be our friend.

Perhaps you rebel at the whole idea of being summed up by a word? If this is the case, sure, I hear you. Yet the fact is that, whether you like it or not, this is the way the world works. Strangers are making assumptions about you, are summing you up over and again. You may as well have some agency in the process.

I didn't have any hesitation about my word when I was first asked about it. It's 'interesting'. I want what I wear to make people think I have things going on (which I do), things to say (which I do), places to go (which I do, be they literal or metaphorical). Now that I have that full-length mirror Carolina Herrera told me every woman should have and use, I always check myself out in it before I leave the front door to check that 'interesting' is indeed how I look.

That said, I also understand where Miuccia Prada is coming from when she talks about her eschewal of the mirror. Sometimes I too am more interested in whether my clothes flatter my internal sense of who I am than my external form. For me too 'what I have in my mind' can be the strongest pull, and I wouldn't have it any other way. To feel interesting is a head thing at least as much as anything else, which is another reason why it is the right word for me.

Some women I talk to tell me they need different words for their personal and professional lives. Again, I understand where they are coming from, but I would argue that it is important to surface your authentic self at work, and that thus it would be good to pin down just the one word if you can. Of course your one word may well have to be reconfigured for different arenas. Rare is the person who can pull off the same look on a Monday morning as on a Saturday night. Find a word that's ambidextrous. There is a way to look 'interesting' – and many other adjectives – for either occasion. Your clothes should be a context-appropriate version of who you are and how you want to be seen. Dressing to reflect who you really are is just as important at work as at the weekend.

That word is going to serve as your north star. But it also helps to have a few other stars by which to navigate. Until shamefully recently both the media and the fashion industry have been so youth obsessed that it has been difficult to find older women who can serve as a style inspiration. Social media has been part of what has changed that. Find people whose style you can identify with, find your tribe, and it can make it easier to work out how to pull off your version of what they do. I am also a big believer in looking around you, in acting like an anthropologist in the field. I am always scoping out what other women wear, and if I see someone who I think is nailing it, I will always go up and compliment her, and maybe find out where she got those boots from, or who is cutting her hair.

Here are just a few of the many women who inspire me.

Iris Apfel, 101

The fact that she needs no introduction shows the power of fashion when it comes to getting yourself seen and keeping yourself relevant. It's not about the date on your birth certificate or the lines on your face. It's about living – and dressing – in joy. 'If you are not pretty you have to develop something else to get around,' Apfel once told me, 'and that serves you well when you get older.'

Emmanuelle Alt, 55

The former editor of French *Vogue* offsets classic minimalism with just the right amount of disco. White blazer plus gold trousers? *Mais oui*.

Cate Blanchett, 53

The actress is the personification of an intelligent fashionista. She never looks try-hard but also sidesteps predictability.

Serena Bute, 62

When the soignée British aristo started to be envious of her kids' track pants she conjured up her own in beautiful silks. With her eponymous label, she pulls off luxurious lounging like no one else.

Lucinda Chambers, 63

No surprise that the woman behind one of my favourite British boutique brands – Colville – should major in the kind of quirkiness that is a life-enhancer.

Inès de la Fressange, 65

If your thing is to look like a Parisienne, then here's your inspiration. The former model manages to make *classique* look youthful rather than staid.

Bella Freud, 61

The designer – and daughter of Lucian – who made slogan knits adult-appropriate walks the line perfectly between cool-kid and grown-up, usually in platform sandals with socks.

Grece Ghanem, 56

This Lebanese microbiologist influencer tends towards Fashion with a capital F. But at her most real-world, she lifts simple, wearable pieces with her inimitable sense of colour.

Clare Hornby, 52

The founder of the British brand Me+Em majors in the kind of effortless contemporaneity that is in her label's DNA.

Renia Jaz, 57

This Polish-born, Newcastle-based influencer – @venswifestyle – is a self-described 'ageism fighter'. One of the ways she fights the good fight is with her joyous – not to mention uncompromising – embrace of cutting-edge fashion.

Diane Keaton, 77

Sometimes this actress is too kooky even for me, yet I love the fact that she always appears so inimitably herself and always seems to be having fun. To my mind, she still looks her best in *Annie-Hall*-style mannish tailoring.

Jenna Lyons, 54

The woman who became famous giving the world just the right mix of masculine and feminine – not to mention the best-ever costume jewellery – is still channelling that J. Crew magic in her own wardrobe.

Rene Macdonald, 52

The designer who came to Britain from Tanzania as a child is the best in the business at delivering classic lines in joyous fabrics, whether it's for her label Lisou or in her daily dress. 'For me Wednesday is a lamé day,' says Macdonald. My kind of blueprint, sorry, goldprint.

Maye Musk, 74

Model-nutritionist-and-mother-of-Elon . . . That's quite some hyphenate existence. Musk got her first cover at 69, and since then the only way has been up. 'Women don't have to slow down as they age,' she writes in her book *A Woman Makes a Plan*. 'I am running like a speeding bullet.' Having met her twice, I can vouch that she is as charming as she is chic.

Michelle Obama, 59

Who says you can't have brains and be into dressing beautifully? There's no better role model for being a formidable fashionista than the former First Lady.

Inge Onsea, 52

Essentiel Antwerp is a go-to brand of mine for style to make you – and everyone else – smile. The woman behind it is predictably brilliant at dopamine dressing.

Miuccia Prada, 73

The Italian designer has been dressing exactly the same for decades, which is to say with an anything but predictable rota of looks that are nothing to do with sexy and everything to do with cerebral. Imagine the chicest librarian ever – that's her.

Linda Rodin, 74

The fashion stylist and former beauty entrepreneur is proof positive that you are never too old for bunches (maybe) and that a bright lipstick is the older woman's ultimate secret weapon. 'I have never thought, "Now I am 40, or 70, I had better dress like this." There was never a separation with the decades,' Rodin recently told me. 'People have sometimes asked me, "Is it appropriate to dress like that?" But I have just never thought in this way.'

Jet Shenkman, 60

There is no better model for Eponine's colourful fit-and-flare frocks in very special fabrics than the boutique label's founder.

Lyn Slater, 68

This American influencer – @iconaccidental – has the second most famous bob in fashion (and hers is grey).

Tilda Swinton, 62

A total sartorial class act. Sometimes looks a tad odd, but never anything other than fabulous.

Petra van Bremen, 62

Hamburg-based model van Bremen gives classicism a contemporary and colourful twist – when she is not channelling streetwear, that is.

Astrid Zeegen, 56

Devon-dwelling Zeegen – @astridiwantyouinmylife – is an advocate for both more (colour and print) and less (stressing about what you should and shouldn't be eating). For which: hurrah!

For me fashion is a female superpower. At this point in history, in Western culture at least, men have so much less room for manoeuvre sartorially – though that is changing, with thanks to Harry Styles among others. To my mind, the sooner men can wear pink, among other things, the better. (The arbitrariness of gendered dress codes is underlined by the fact that pink was for a boy until the beginning of the last century.)

In the meantime, let's embrace everything that clothes can offer us women. Men who want to stay within the mainstream have barely any choices to make about what they wear. As a woman you can shapeshift day by day. You can sport mannish tailoring one minute, a floral dress the next. I love the freedom I have to pick and choose how I want to garb myself, and to influence how I feel as a result.

Because clothes do change the way you feel. One of the most striking anecdotes I have ever heard about the power of clothes comes from the charity Smart Works. It helps women who have been struggling to find a job, women who are typically referred to them by other charities, job centres, prisons and the NHS. What's universal among these women is a lack of confidence. Even when they have gone for jobs for which they have the right qualifications, they still don't get them.

The Smart Works volunteers give them coaching on how to succeed at interview. They also ask each woman how she would like to look for her interview, and then – using rails of donated clothes – set out to deliver the closest approximation that they can. According to the charity's co-founder Juliet Hughes-Hallett, 'When they stand in front of the mirror in their new outfit, it's a real hair-standing-on-end moment. You can see them thinking, "My God, this might actually be possible." It is like they have put on a suit of armour.'

I am not suggesting that you need to armour yourself for ageing, rather that you need to open up your fashion choices, perhaps more than you ever have before; to be *less* armoured, if anything, or at least to be armoured in a different way. You need to surface yourself more than you may have felt able to do when you were younger.

To dress youthfully is both to feel youthful and to be seen as youthful, just as, in that Harvard experiment that took a group of men back to a version of their 1950s past, they began to behave and feel like younger men.

In their 2012 essay 'Enclothed Cognition' the psychologists Adam D Galinsky and Hajo Adam talk of 'the systematic influence that clothes have on a wearer's psychological processes'. That influence is the result of 'two independent factors', they continue, 'the symbolic meaning of clothes and the physical experience of wearing them'.

The pair conducted a series of experiments which, I imagine you will be unsurprised to learn, didn't focus on the impact of wearing a Snoopy T-shirt with a suit. But still. I'll let Galinsky and Adam take it from here. 'A pre-test found that a lab coat is generally associated with attentiveness and carefulness,' they wrote. 'We therefore predicted that wearing a lab coat would increase performance on attention-related tasks. In Experiment 1, physically wearing a lab coat increased selective attention compared to not wearing a lab coat. In Experiments 2 and 3, wearing a lab coat described as a doctor's coat increased sustained attention compared to wearing a lab coat described as a painter's coat . . .'

Enough about lab coats! Let's have a look at some easy ways to freshen your wardrobe. So you have your word. Now have a proper look at what you own already. Find an empty Saturday afternoon if you can. I am an advocate for taking everything off your rails and out of your drawers and sorting it into piles, ideally on a spare bed, in a room on which you can close the door.

There is the pile of clothes that already personify that word you chose for yourself. There is the pile of clothes that may not personify said word, but that will work well with those that do. (It's not that everything I own ticks the 'interesting' box, for example, but if it doesn't, I know that it foregrounds what does.) There is also the pile of clothes that aren't working on either front, and/or that may no longer fit your body or your lifestyle, or have become tatty, or – and this is usually a telltale sign – have not been worn for a year or more.

Try on as much as you need in order to work out which pieces should be in which pile. Put that full-length mirror to good use. Take your time. Be open. Be experimental. Have fun. And then stop. And shut the door.

Cue Sunday afternoon. Go back to your piles. Focus on pile number three first, the one full of items that aren't currently delivering. Get rid of as much of it as you can, the only exceptions being items with sentimental value, items that you might realistically (realistically!) fit back into in six months, and anything that, even if it doesn't quite fit your brief, makes you look and/or feel great.

Go through piles one and two again, just to make sure you got it right first time. Check too that you don't have any unnecessary duplicates. Of course brands want you to buy more, but the savviest fashion folk edit, edit, edit, having – for example – two top-notch and differently styled pairs of jeans rather than ten. Be particularly critical when it comes to old shoes and bags, too. There is nothing that more quickly dates you – or transforms you – than your accessories. Get rid of everything that doesn't serve you, perhaps by selling it online, or taking it to your local charity shop or clothes bank, or passing it on to friends or family. Start to think too about what you are missing, and might need to invest in. (More on that in a minute.)

Put everything that you think is working for you back on your rails, in your drawers and on your shelves.

And give yourself a year to do a further edit. So often we have ideas about what we think we wear that don't actually stack up with what we reach for in reality. Every time you take something out of your wardrobe and wear it over that year, return it to the rail with the coat hanger turned the other way. By the end of the year your wardrobe will bear witness to what you do and don't use.

It's trickier to enact the same truth-reveal with the clothes you keep in drawers and shelves. If you get rid of enough in the first place you will hopefully find yourself with at least one empty drawer and shelf. Each time you wear something, move it to that drawer or shelf afterwards. That may empty up another drawer or shelf that you can then fill with more items you actually wear. Eventually you should end up with at least one drawer and shelf of things that you don't. You know now what happens next with that!

When it comes to new acquisitions, there are certain pieces that I think are instant youthifiers. Footwear first. A pair of classic white trainers, for example, will change up everything from a trouser suit to a floral dress. A pair of ankle boots – perhaps a chunky Chelsea style, or something a bit more fine – will also modernise pretty much everything. If you can stretch to a pair of knee-high boots too, they are great with a dress all winter. (I swear by Russell & Bromley boots, not to mention its flatform trainers which deliver a bit of leg-lengthening lift.) If you are up for heels, go for an all-day height – there is nothing more ageing than not being able to walk effortlessly – and check out the classic-with-a-twist styles on offer at brands such as Aeyde or Arket.

A casual jacket, perhaps a so-called shacket, or shirt jacket, will transform that same frock, or look just as good with tailored trousers as with jeans. Indeed, mixing and matching items that would once have seemed incongruous – essentially pairing smart with street – immediately looks contemporary. A fine cashmere hoodie worn under a blazer would be another case in point. Or a leather biker jacket over a chiffon frock.

One more approach is to buy a single item that does the hybridising for you, such as a pair of well-cut satin track pants that are cool as well as feminine, or a dress with athleisure-style zip detailing. Me+Em is the brand I return to time and again for clothes that are subtly tweaked in this way, and that are also designed to work together, so you can gradually building-block your way, season by season.

What's great these days, not to mention a tad ironic, is that many of the clothes that are in with the young are extrapolations of what, once upon a time, would have been worn more by older women. At time of writing the high street is full of midi dresses with sleeves; of blouses and blazers. And never have there been so many options, so many different ways to dress.

Think too about layering, and in ways that are – and, yes, I am going to use that word again – unexpected. This is another route to appearing – warning: fashion-industry terminology incoming! – relevant. A long-sleeved tee peeping out under a day dress, for example, with a knitted tank layered over it, and perhaps a biker jacket on top; even – in the depths of winter – an overcoat on top of that. This is the way to navigate different temperatures day to day, not to mention day to night, as well as to find your way to a trans-seasonal wardrobe that will work for you all year round. You can simply layer up or down, depending on the weather.

Arket is a great brand for layerable pieces that sit at the sweet spot between classic and contemporary. Playing with different weights and textures – mohair with silk, leather with wool – also looks modern.

Colour is another route to making yourself manifest. As Henri Matisse once said, 'With colour one obtains an energy which seems to stem from witchcraft.' It gets you seen on the most literal level. There is a reason why it is often deployed in the animal kingdom to attract a mate. It also adds interest to the simple lines that tend to look more modern. Fussy tends to make you appear fussy. A clean yet colourful silhouette is an effortless way to get noticed.

I have always regularly worn colour, but I would only ever wear one piece at a time. That coral jacket would be paired with black trousers and top, for example. Nothing wrong with that. It absolutely does the job. And how – as I have already said – I pity poor men for not feeling able to lift their look or put a pep in their step by way of some colour. On days when I look and feel bad 50, not good 50, I know I can fake it to make it. I need never look grey, even though my hair is.

These days I often wear ensembles that consist of several different colours. It looks so 21st century. One easy way in is to embrace the so-called tone-on-tone approach, pairing two different shades of the same hue, like a purple and a lilac, or a pink and a red. Another route is to mix colours that are opposite on the colour wheel, such as blue and orange, or red and green. Easier still is to pick one multi-hue item that does the work for you.

Once you get braver – as I have over time – you may find yourself wanting to push the envelope more and more. I have found that adding a third colour into the mix usually busts any rules about what goes with what. These days, if I like what I see in that aforementioned mirror of mine, I go with it!

There are a few tricks to ascertaining what colours work best with your skin undertone. Hold a piece of pure white paper next to your make-up-less face. When you look in the mirror, how does your skin appear? If you have a cool skin undertone you will look rosy, pink, red or blue. If you have a warm skin undertone it will be yellow, green or light brown. If you appear grey or ashen you probably have a neutral skin undertone. This test should work whatever your ethnicity. If you are struggling to make your mind up, you can also try the jewellery route. Cool types tend to suit silver jewellery best, warm types gold, and neutral can go with either.

In terms of the colours that will flatter your skin, the key is to stick with those that are related. This means that cools suit cool shades that make you think of winter or the sea, such as blues, blue-greens, purples, magentas and blue-based reds. Strong neutrals such as black, bright white, navy and good greys also work. Warms, on the other hand, are better in yellows, oranges, browns, yellow-greens, orange-based reds and softer neutrals such as creams, taupes and gentle greys. Neutral skin undertones tend to have more latitude. Some can get away with almost anything, colour wise, while others need to avoid colours that overwhelm them – picking a blue that's soft rather than electric, for example, or an off-white rather than a pure white.

Bear in mind, too, that if there is a colour you love but that doesn't love you, you may well be able to get away with it, as long as you don't wear it next to your skin. A bright handbag is a great way to pull this off. It's the ultimate mood-lifter to have a bag in a colour you adore, and I have found from experience that precisely because a bag doesn't in theory go with anything, it tends to go with everything. I also think a small crossbody – or even a luxe leather belt-bag slung across the body bandolier style – immediately youthifies your look more than a shoulder bag or tote. The last thing you want is to appear in any way encumbered or uptight.

I have become much braver with pattern, as well. When I was younger I never really wore it. More recently I set out on the same path I went with colour many years previously. I would wear a single patterned piece, and keep everything else plain around it. I started with another one of my beloved statement jackets. Next stop was a dress that clash-matched two different patterns for me, floral in the main but with stripey inserts. Again, it's that contemporising unexpectedness that is so potent.

Now I sometimes clash-match two different patterns myself. One way to make this fly is to pair two contrasting designs that are united by their colour palette, perhaps a green and white check with a green and white floral. Another is to pick contrasting versions of the same print, perhaps a houndstooth or a polka dot in two contrasting colours and scales.

Also worth factoring in when it comes to the power of pattern is the modernity that comes with wearing traditionally 'winter' patterns on summer fabrics – like animal print or houndstooth on silk – or a 'summery' print on a winter-weight textile. My much-loved wool overcoat is printed with a tropical floral.

Embellishment is another way to add interest. A bit of embroidery here or a sequin there on an otherwise clean silhouette, or a sliver of lace or pussy-bow flourish can work wonders. Essentiel Antwerp is the best I have found at this, and at larger-than-life brooches and necklaces that can add *joie de vivre* to even the plainest of black ensembles.

On the subject of jewellery, I love the modernised baroque pearls at homegrown brands such as Monica

Vinader and Completedworks. Don't wear your mother's pearls: too dating. But channel the complexion-burnishing magic that pearls have always offered up. And consider, too, the magic wand that can be waved by a so-called curation of chain necklaces, perhaps with a locket or two, like those from Kirstie Le Marque or Missoma.

Indeed, jewellery is a great way to change the way you present without any kind of wardrobe overhaul. There is no one better at this than Iris Apfel, she of the goggle glasses and huge necklaces. She once told me she learned everything she knows from her mother. 'She was extremely chic. She worshipped at the altar of the accessory: she could do more tricks with a scarf than anyone I have ever met. She taught me that style is about attitude. It has nothing to do with money.'

Attitude. It's where we began this chapter. It seems only right that it is where we should end it. Whatever you wear, own it. Be it. Enjoy it. Here's one email I have received from a reader of *The Times* who has followed my regular exhortations to do just that: 'Reading your fashion articles has woken up my curiosity and I have enjoyed experimenting *massively*. Now as I approach my 60th birthday, I am happy in size 14 and feeling good about my clothes and unapologetic re. massive pants.' Here's to *that*!

If you are changing your look, the people who know you may be a little surprised at first. It's all good. You are coming into yourself: revealing the true you like never before. Besides, I have learned from experience that, if you keep on showing up – wearing pink, or a biker jacket, or indeed a pink biker jacket, or whatever else it may be – that surprise soon fades.

To dress to reveal who you really are is to pull off precisely that. To dress your best is to come one step closer to being your best.

9

Family, Old and New

Growing older offers us the chance to find that differentiation from others that can be so hard to pin down in the first decades of our life; to interrogate who we are in relation only to ourselves. Much of what I have written about so far has pertained to finding and expanding that self. Now is also the time to take stock not only of who you are, but of the people around you, of what does and doesn't work about the relationships you have with them, and to reconfigure accordingly.

Becoming more clear-sighted about ourselves gives us the opportunity in turn to spring-clean our closest relationships, whether with family or friends. Because let's not underestimate the degree to which we will always exist in the context of relationships. Acknowledging that we are a self-defining entity is essential to finding a sense of both purpose and contentment. Yet our wider milieu is important, too. Besides, dusting out our friendship closet helps us to come full circle in consolidating who we really are.

It is only as you grow older that you come to understand how life – other people's as well as your own – is like a novel. To watch a relative's or an old friend's chapters unfold over the years is both a privilege and a learning experience. But the most useful learning will come from flicking through your own backstory. Look for patterns. Do you have a tendency to be drawn to friendships that don't serve you in some way? Do you have patterns of behaviour in relationships that aren't working for you? Do you end up in a particular role over and again even though it is one that drives you mad?

Sometimes what you find may surprise you. You may be distracted by extraneous information. In my twenties, for example, I had two friends whom I struggled with in different ways. They couldn't stand each other. For years, the fact that they didn't like each other stopped me from seeing that they were both versions of the same thing, both trying to control me. Indeed, their similarity was probably precisely why they didn't get on.

When I finally joined the control-freak dots I was better able to sidestep anyone similar going forward. Repetitious tendencies tend not to happen by accident but to be the result of subconscious design, often rooted in your childhood. What maps are you using when it comes to your interactions with other people? Get rid of the ones that are taking you to the wrong destination!

We are going to talk about romantic partners in the next chapter. This chapter is about the other close relationships that can help to shape your life for good or ill. Remember that Lao Tzu quote about thoughts becoming words, words becoming actions, actions becoming habits, and habits determining both who you are and, eventually, your destiny? I think it might also legitimately encompass the people you have in your life, because they too will have an impact on your thoughts, words, actions . . . and so it goes on. The Buddha said, 'We are what we think.' Jean Anthelme

Brillat-Savarin, a 19th-century French gastronome, came up with something along the lines of 'You are what you eat.'

I would argue that we are also who we know. Who you spend time with inevitably plays a part in shaping who you become. So you want the good ones: the ones who make you more rather than less; the ones who make you laugh, not cry; the ones with whom you can be serious but also silly; the ones who make you think, maybe challenging your beliefs or assumptions, but who also help you to not think, to just be; the ones who give you things (great experiences, food for thought, joy), but also leave you feeling unburdened.

Research would suggest that the more we are socially hooked up, the better we will age and the longer we will live. It's one more of those balancing acts that is a defining feature not just of getting older but of being alive, that *we* need to complete *ourselves*, but that we can then augment that self through positive connections with others.

Two shared characteristics of the so-called 'blue zones' of the world – where a higher than average number of people live longer than average – have been defined as 'family' and 'social engagement'. In their book *Successful Aging* (1998), John W Rowe and Robert L Kahn, American medical professors, observe that 'Connectedness is pivotal to successful aging as it can influence both physical and emotional health.' Or as E M Forster famously exhorted in *Howard's End*, 'Only connect.'

As a species, *Homo sapiens* is defined by our capacity to do just that. As is noted by Stephanie Cacioppo, the author of *Wired for Love: A Neuroscientist's Journey Through Romance, Loss and the Essence of Human Connection* (2022), it was our social skills that allowed us to supersede Neanderthals 70,000 years ago. 'The Neanderthals were fearsome competition: bigger, stronger, with better vision and brains that may have been slightly larger than those of humans. But the neural architecture of the Neanderthals and *Homo sapiens* differed in important ways. The Neanderthals had more space dedicated to vision and motor skills – they were ideal physical warriors. But the *Homo sapiens* were ideal social warriors: they could understand the intentions of others, they could consider a choice from two sides, they learned quickly from their mistakes.'

So we humans are wired to be sociable. The problem is that some of the wiring can be faultily installed. When we are growing up it can be challenging to distinguish between who we are and who the people around us want us to be. In our early years there is so much information coming at us, so much noise, it can be hard to turn down the volume on what isn't useful to us and turn up the volume on what is. That impacts upon the kind of relationships in which we find ourselves. Whether they are the apparently non-negotiable bonds of family, or the more negotiable ones of friendship or romance, they may be formulated to someone else's guidelines, not our own.

As children we also learn that relationships tend to be about power, who has it and who doesn't. Most of our earliest relationships are with those who are older than us, and so are unequal, with us as the junior partner. No wonder so many of us, when we find ourselves with a younger sibling, immediately transform into a despot. (Sorry, Fran!) No wonder our schools and workplaces are full of bullies. No wonder tyrannical husbands and wives, girlfriends and boyfriends are two a penny.

So how do we find the blueprints for relationships that aren't about power, either the wielding of it or the subjugation in the face of it? Many of us don't. For me growing older has given me the wherewithal to forge relationships of all sorts that have nothing to do with power. When I was younger I didn't have the discernment even to ascertain that this might be a goal, never mind the capacity to enact it.

I began with my sister, though it shamefully took me until my twenties to do so. Rewiring how Fran and I were as siblings was a true through-the-looking-glass moment for me. To express your vulnerability to someone, your not-knowingness, and to do so with humility, can be – ironically – one of the most empowering experiences imaginable.

It was with Fran that I took my first steps in true openness, and in forging a relationship that was entirely without competitiveness, *Schadenfreude* or smallness of any kind. It was this that paved the way to me finding friendships of true equality, genuine two-way streets, with people of all ages and from all walks of life. My life has been transformed as a result.

You can refresh your existing connections just by approaching them differently. I was the one who enacted the change in the relationship with my sister because, at that point, I, as the senior party, had the wherewithal to do so. She shapeshifted almost instantaneously. As Nikola Tesla, the Serbian-American inventor whom some credit with the invention of the radio, once said, 'If you want to find the secrets of the universe, think in terms of energy, frequency and vibration.' Change your energy around someone, change your frequency, your vibration, and they will, probably entirely unconsciously, change theirs.

Another idea is to do something new together. Take them along to something you love, or go along to something they love, or pick something that neither of you has ever done but always quite fancied the idea of. Bring up topics of conversation that you have never talked about, or haven't touched upon for years; discuss the things that really matter to you. Or bring up the things that don't matter at all, but that make you laugh.

Having fun is important. Making each other laugh; being silly; channelling your inner child. The most striking aspect of the wonderful documentary *Mission: Joy – Finding Happiness in Troubled Times* (2021) is how the Dalai Lama and the since-departed Desmond Tutu spend most of their time together mucking around like small boys. Speaking personally, I was delighted to note when watching this programme that a love of mickey-taking evidently does not get in the way of spiritual transcendence.

You can woo a friend, or be wooed by a friend, just as you can a romantic partner, and it can be an enriching experience for you both. You can draw new boundaries, too. Every relationship is a sum of two parts. If the sum isn't working for you any more, you can change your part – the role you do or don't take, the ways you do or don't respond – and see how the overall sum changes in turn.

Of course, it may be that some aspects of the equation work and others don't. That's fine, as long as overall the good outweighs the bad. If the sum still doesn't add up, however, and it's a friend rather than family, you can and should walk away from them. If it's family, it's infinitely harder, but engaging on your own terms, while operating from a place of compassion, is key. Sometimes even with family you may need to disengage, if not entirely then partially.

It's like that instruction they always give on an aeroplane: in the event of a crash you should put your own mask on before you put on anyone else's. If someone won't let you put your mask on, or even worse – and this applies to the father of one dear friend – keeps trying to pull it off when it's on, then it makes sense to at the very least limit the time you spend with them, the headspace you give to them and the influence you accord to them. That same idea of a noticing bracelet that we spoke about as a means of pulling ourselves into the present can also be used to pull ourselves *away* from negative thoughts pertaining to another person, or indeed anything else.

Luckily, these days you can make your own family. I have two brothers who aren't blood, and at least half a dozen sisters. I also have several children who aren't, in fact, mine!

I would argue that growing older should be a time when you inject some fresh blood, too: individuals who reflect – and amplify – exactly who you are now, not a version of yourself from decades earlier. A couple of my aforementioned sisters, for example, I met only in the last few years. So many of our relationships tend to be a matter of circumstance, forged out of a particular time (being a new mother, say) or place (colleagues or college friends are the most obvious examples of that). This is especially the case in those busy decades in which you are making your way in the world. When you are older, you can seek out new connections based on commonalities that have a different kind of depth.

Theories of so-called social capital explore the idea of 'bonded' groups and 'bridging' groups, the former a closed shop (the people you work with or went to college with, for example), the latter open to anyone who wants to join. One reason why it seems to have become harder to meet new people in real life – be it a would-be friend or a romantic partner – is that 21st-century life is organised more around bonded groups than bridging groups than it was a generation or two ago. Sociologists say it takes an average of 50 hours to make a casual friend and about 200 hours to form a close bond with someone.

To seek out a community engaged in something you enjoy – a bridging group – is a fantastic way to find new friends. For me that has been yoga. Just one of the aspects I have been surprised by – more than that, delighted – is the intergenerational nature of my resultant friendships.

Maye Musk is typically wise on the power of good, not to mention diverse, friendships. 'If you learn anything from me,' she writes in her book, 'let it be this: don't be afraid of aging, and mix with friends who are not afraid of aging. Have fun with your friends, of all ages, who like you because you are fascinating, interesting, intelligent, confident, and maybe stylish (in your mind). Listen to others, be good to others, no matter their ages. If someone tells you you're too old, especially if you are dating that person, say goodbye.'

Among my closest friends now are women decades

younger and decades older than me. To hear what someone in their twenties or sixties has to say about the world is not just fascinating but extremely useful. It keeps me mentally supple. It keeps me open-minded. It keeps me empathetic.

My partner Chris – a 40-something skateboarder – has had the same experience. He hangs out with skaters in their twenties through to their sixties. He and his older skater friends often joke about how people tell them they are 'too old' to skate. Why? Why do we still have these outmoded notions about what is or isn't a suitable activity?

We have changed our thinking around clothes, the world now full of retirees in jeans and trainers, once the uniform of youth. Now we need to do the same with hobbies. Chris tells me that several times he has met men at his skate park who are there to watch their young children, and who tell him somewhat sadly that they used to skate before they got 'too old'. Chris always invites them to borrow his board. Twenty minutes later they are back, eyes shining. Most of them now turn up with their own board each week, and have a whale of a time. What a great thing to model for their kids, skating the bowl alongside them, a personification of the fact that you are never too old, if you just make up your mind not to be.

When it comes to my younger friends in particular, I gain enormous validation from the degree to which I am able to help them with the perspectives I have had more time to develop. A friend who is not only older but open is one of the most precious friends you can have. Remember that grandmother hypothesis we talked about in Chapter 3. As you grow older, your potential value to others is immense, whether or not you happen to have grandchildren.

One notable feature of this period of life for many of us is that it is when children leave home. I don't have children myself. However, what I have witnessed among my most sane friends is that this is the ultimate example of saying goodbye to say hello. It's a loss, certainly, but also a gain, an occasion to take a fresh look at who you are and what you want, and to recalibrate your life accordingly. It's an opportunity first and foremost for you to live for you again. 'The only symptom of empty-nest syndrome,' according to Daniel Gilbert, professor of psychology at Harvard University, 'is smiling.' That's an over-simplification, certainly, but it's an over-simplification that can be helpful.

What hobby and/or ambition have you put on hold because of Cyril Connolly's 'pram in the hall'? Many friends, female ones in particular, have talked to me about 'losing' themselves – their word not mine – in the process of bringing up children. Wonderful as motherhood may be, it's the ultimate role in which to be cast, a role which is by definition a supporting one. Once your children have grown, you can take on a leading role once again.

This is also the moment for you to do due diligence on the nature of your parent-child bond. Is there any aspect of it that might helpfully be tweaked? Remember that Hoffman Process conception of parenting as being akin to a game of Chinese whispers. The new-found spaciousness that comes with a child leaving home may shed light on any irrelevant freighting that you have unwittingly bestowed on them, especially if you are looking at what you were freighted with before them. And here is your best chance yet, if you haven't done so already, to forge a relationship between equals, one which, apart from anything else, is going to be far more interesting for you than one that's predicated on any notion of teacher and student, superior and inferior.

Dorothy Rowe is among those who have gone as far as to declare that there exists 'a mutual antipathy' between youth and age. In *Time on Our Side* she puts this down to the fact that 'The idea that children are people in their own right, not merely objects owned by their parents, has never been popular, not even today.'

It is the disempowerment many of us feel as children, Rowe argues, that prompts us subconsciously to enact a kind of vengeful disempowerment on our parents when they become older. When I first came across her thesis I thought it seemed a bit much. Now I wonder if she might be onto something. Either way, now is the moment, if you haven't done so already, to transform your son or daughter into a friend and ally.

When I asked my 18-year-old goddaughter Edie recently what makes a good parent, she wisely replied,

'It's about continuing to live your own life. That way you don't end up trying to live your child's.' Her parents – my friends – had never made that mistake, she said, but so many of her friends' parents had, and were continuing to do so. Guess which kind of parent is going to adjust more easily when their child leaves home? But it's never too late to adapt.

Your child isn't your responsibility any more. You shouldn't be telling them what to do. You should be listening to and enjoying what they are. It's a genuine two-way street at last, and you are most definitely not in charge of traffic control. What a liberation. Now you can sit back and read *their* novel in a more relaxed way. What will their next chapter be? And the one after that? There can be no more fascinating read for a parent, which is not to say it will be entirely without future trials.

Another familial challenge many of us will face in this period of our lives is helping our own parent or parents deal with illness or infirmity. If you are in the lucky position of enjoying a straightforward relationship with your parent, then this can represent a comparatively straightforward chance to serve; to pay them back – in the best sense – for all that they did for you. There will be the practical and organisational hardship of being there for and helping an ill person; there will be the emotional hardship of watching a person you love suffer; and for the growing numbers of us having to deal with dementia, there will be the existential hardship of losing the person, to a greater or lesser degree, before you actually lose them. However, the equation at the heart of it all – in your heart – will make some kind of sense.

Far more problematic to negotiate is the act of caring for a parent with whom you have struggled, or indeed still struggle. As with all these balancing acts that we must negotiate in life, only you know what the true path is for you.

Either way you may need to check in with what you realistically can and can't do, especially if this is a medium- to long-term situation. Some kind of mindfulness practice – whether you think of it as meditation or just sitting in silence – should, if you keep on showing up for it, eventually provide you with some clarity.

Think too of that aeroplane-mask analogy. You have to look after yourself in order to be able to look after others. To martyr yourself indefinitely for someone else serves no one. Certainly, you don't want to have regrets about what you did or didn't do. Yet putting your own life on hold and, as all too often becomes the case, jeopardising your health, is something to be regretted too. My goddaughter's words about what makes a good parent can also be applied to being a child. You have to live your own life, not someone else's.

Whatever the obstacles, keep in mind the words of the Greek Stoic philosopher Epictetus: 'See difficulty as an opportunity to prove yourself.' What's hard for you is often – with the right attitude – a nudge towards expansion, acceleration, learning things that you wouldn't have learned otherwise, facing up to things that you might otherwise have continued to look away from.

Bearing witness to the end of someone's life forces us to lock eyes with that ultimate facelessness that is death, to turn towards not just our parent's mortality but our own. In a culture that defaults to looking away from death, it's no wonder this is a challenging time for many of us.

Belief in an afterlife or another reincarnated life gave meaning to this experience for millennia, but many of us now live without that succour. When I bore witness to the devastation wrought on a friend – a rationalist to his core – by the death of his father, I found myself wishing that he did have some kind of belief system to help him through. Whatever your position on the idea of an afterlife or lives, it certainly works as a placebo, and in that alone there is surely a value.

However, you don't need belief to make death a better experience for all concerned. We as a culture are obsessed with not-dying, and fearful of dying, a state of mind that infects the very thing it seeks to disinfect us against. 'Death,' as the Bosnian novelist Mesa Selimovic wrote in *Death and the Dervish* (1996), 'is the only thing that we know will befall us.' So why not focus instead on doing it well? A good death, or as good a death as can be managed under the circumstances, is one of the greatest gifts you can give to anyone you love.

The vision laid out in Claire Montanaro's book

Spiritual Wisdom: Practical Spirituality for People Today (2008) is one of the most useful I have found, just a few elements of which I will touch upon here. 'All the major civilisations have had their own ways of marking death, some of them intensely profound,' she writes. 'In the Western world now, the process can be distorted by medical interference and logistical prioritisation so that the dying process often is managed by drugs in a noisy environment where the patient is treated as an object not a person.'

Montanaro, who works as a spiritual teacher and channeller, advocates if possible initiating a conversation with your loved one long beforehand about what a good death might look like to them, whether they would like, for example, to die at home, or in a clinic or hospital. If it's the former, a charity such as Marie Curie can offer help if and when required. If it is you facing death, whether near or far, it is for you to initiate that conversation with those to whom you are closest.

Whichever side of the fence you are on, when both you and your loved ones become aware that the time is approaching, this is the moment to pin down specifics.

'Is there any music they [or you] would like in their room, special flowers, a candle, anyone they would wish to be present – or not?'

At the moment of death, continues Montanaro, it is important not to impede your loved one's passing, but instead to understand 'the importance of allowing your loved one to leave the Earth plane when <u>they</u> are ready and not to try to keep them with you longer than they would wish'. [Montanaro's underlining.] Instead those assembled should 'pray for your loved one's highest good and well-being, not, specifically, their continuing survival in body'. The act of praying can, of course, equate simply to a peaceful, directed form of contemplation, a spiritual act in the broadest sense, rather than anything to do with religion per se.

The ultimate goal, says Montanaro, is to make death 'as uplifting and beautiful an occasion as it can possibly be'. She writes about how those she has counselled in changing their approach and involvement in a loved one's death have told her 'how adopting these procedures helped . . . their grieving process enormously'.

There will still be grief when your loved one is gone,

of course. And that is if you are lucky. There may also be additional, more toxic feelings such as guilt and anger. If it is primarily grief that you are feeling, then give thanks for that. It means that you have loved and been loved. It means that you have shared so much with that person. Do not deny the sadness you feel at them passing, but try also to surface happiness about the fact that they were in your life in the first place.

This will take time. Negativity and positivity will dance together day by day, the former probably leading the latter across the floor for a while. But if you keep checking in with the good, and giving thanks, the moving landscape that is grief will be illuminated by the occasional shaft of sunlight far more quickly. The human condition is one of *chiaroscuro*. The *chiaro* can only be foregrounded if there is also *scuro*.

The final chapter of that novel which is someone's life can, if you just have the eyes to see it, be as beautiful in its own way as the first, perhaps more so. If it is not, however – if your parent is dying with regrets, for example – there is precious learning in that for you. Your last few decades should be lived in the consciousness that your life will come to an end, said consciousness begetting not morbidity but rather the desire to live and love as fully as possible. The potency of *chiaroscuro* again. The importance of joy.

10

True Romance

Are you in a long-term relationship? Are you single? Are you dating? Are you in a new relationship? Are you in the process of disentangling yourself from a relationship? That your answer could be yes to any of these five different questions is in itself, at our stage in life, a revolution. It didn't used to be the case.

In the last decade I have been in all of the above categories at one point or another. To be single, then not-single, then single, then not-single again as a fully fledged adult has been one of the most interesting and valuable experiences of my life to date, which is not to say that it hasn't at times also been hard. I have learned so much about myself, and the world. I have also had a lot of fun.

Mere decades ago an older person's romantic status was considered to be a closed book. You were married (well done) or widowed (poor you) or a spinster (what a disaster). It's just one illustration of how bogus such thinking is that I had some of my unhappiest times towards the end of a long-term relationship that was a marriage in all but name (not well done at all), and that I had some of my happiest times when I was a spinster (sic) in my forties (the opposite of a disaster). One of the greatest gifts of my adult life has been the years I spent on my own, not that it necessarily always felt like that in the moment.

Today, we are freer than ever to choose not to be in a relationship, or to exit one that doesn't serve us. There may be some around us who still judge, but many of those will be secretly jealous of the freedom and adventure that singletons tend to be able to access more easily. I know I could sometimes be that quietly envious coupled-up person once upon a time.

On the other hand, if we *are* in a relationship, or would like to be in one again, we also have more opportunity than ever to formulate one that works for who we are now, whether that entails a recalibration, large or small, of a partnership we have been in for many years, or forging a new relationship.

Would I have been sounding quite so positive about all this when I was scrolling through Bumble on, say, a dark Thursday evening in December three years ago? Possibly not. But, a couple of nights later, on a date with someone dashingly inappropriate, I would have. And I would have, too, on all those many occasions of comparatively recent singledom when I have felt so entirely me, so entirely free, so entirely and directly connected to the world without anyone else getting in the way.

Positive is what I am today, too, now that I am with someone I met on – of all the unlikely platforms – Tinder, someone who suits the woman I have become, with a lot of work and learning, at 50. At least as importantly for me I know, too, that if I were to become single again, I would be able to embrace the many upsides once more.

If we find our right place in the world, and our right people, we need never be defined by whether we are or aren't in a relationship. When I found myself single at 34, after 14 years with my college sweetheart, many of the people around me were as confused by my new-found status as I was. I had been one thing, now I was another. What I had done, I now understand, is allowed my identity to meld into another's. Who was I as only half of that whole we had created together?

These days I have learned how to be complete in and of myself. The people who know and love me couldn't give a damn what is or isn't happening in my romantic life. (Although in the recent past they have loved to live vicariously when things got exciting.) And my other half loves me precisely because I – like him – am already complete. He augments me, and I augment him. There is no completing going on.

The 19th-century American essayist Ralph Waldo Emerson once wisely observed that 'We must be our own before we can be another's.' It's my singleton years that have made me my own to a degree that I didn't find possible previously. When I was growing up, I was too influenced by parents, and authority more generally; too desirous to listen to other people, to be a good girl.

My formative romantic relationships tended – surprise, surprise – to follow a similar theme.

They also inevitably drew on the models for a relationship that I had witnessed in my life to date, none of which were right for me. We aren't taught how to love or be loved. We pick things up as we go along. And a lot of it isn't that helpful, whether it's extrapolated from life or literature. Indeed, it's remarkable, given the degree to which love stories fill the metaphorical airwaves, how few of them are actually useful for those of us who want to learn to do it better. Good love, wise love, love that truly lasts, never mind grows, is rare to find, and thus difficult to bear witness to.

The late novelist Elizabeth Jane Howard, who was three times divorced, summed the situation up perfectly for me when she appeared on *Desert Island Discs* in 1995, when she was in her seventies: 'I believe in love now but in a very different way. I think then I believed it was something that happened to you, and I think now it's something that comes about out of who you are to begin with. I don't think I was fit for love really . . . I think really good love, I am not even saying great love, is actually relatively rare . . . People talk about it a lot, which means the idea is that because everybody could fall in love, or have love, they think everybody does. I think this is not true. I think it is a remarkable gift. And if it is something you hold very dearly, all you can do is get yourself ready to be that sort of person . . .'

So how do we ready ourselves? How do we get better at loving, whether we are in a relationship or not? Pretty much everything you need to know is in a wonderful little book called *The Art of Loving* (1957) by Erich Fromm. OK, so Fromm is not so hot on how to manage the dating apps, what with him having died in 1980. But if you are looking to give those a try, I will be giving you the ultimate cheat sheet shortly. What Fromm is great on is the fabric that makes up a loving relationship, the cloth you weave together.

His basic point is that loving is a verb, a thing that you do; more than that, a thing that you practise. 'Love is an activity,' he writes, 'not a passive affect; it is "standing in", not a "falling for". In the most general way, the active character of love can be described by stating that love is primarily *giving*, not receiving.' (All italics are Fromm's in this and the ensuing quotes.) Love is also 'not primarily a relationship to a specific person; it is an *attitude*, an *orientation of character* which determines the relatedness of a person to the world as a whole, not towards one "object" of love.'

I once interviewed a woman who ran an expensive bespoke dating agency. She said that in her extensive experience she had come to the conclusion that if someone found the right person when they were 27 or younger it was more good luck than good management. Most people didn't know themselves well enough, and were still works in progress to too great a degree, to get it right at that age. I definitely got it wrong.

She also spoke about how a common cause of relationship failure is that givers tend to pick takers, and vice versa. That serves the taker perfectly well, needless to say, but it can go wrong when the giver suddenly finds themselves at a place in their life where they need to take – perhaps due to bereavement or the loss of a job – and realise that they are with someone who is less able to give. The woman at the dating agency always tried to match a giver with another giver, she said. Something else I got wrong until embarrassingly recently. Actions do speak louder than words. The world is full of lovers who talk the talk, but far fewer walk the walk.

A successful long-term relationship is about giving to someone, showing up for someone over and again; about remaining interested and engaged in who they are today, and who they are evolving towards becoming tomorrow, rather than just assuming they are the same person they were when you first met.

Yet at the same time a proper partnership is about maintaining your individuality, not subsuming yourself into someone else's. 'Mature *love* is *union under the condition of preserving one's integrity, one's individuality,*' says Fromm. '*Love is an active power in man*; a power which breaks through the walls which separate man from his fellow men, which unites him with others; love makes him overcome the sense of isolation and separateness, yet it permits him to be himself, to retain his integrity. In love the paradox occurs that two beings become one and yet remain two.'

How do we make love last? 'By finding novelty every day and being curious about your significant other,' according to Stephanie Cacioppo.

'Love goes wrong when we forget to tell people who we are and forget to ask who they are,' agrees Susie Orbach.

Cacioppo warns about the 'two-year slump', that point at which the novelty starts to wear off, which can be more of a relationship threat than the far better known seven-year itch. 'If people feel they are growing apart, knowing a little bit more about their brains could help. What they are experiencing is not necessarily their fault; there are biological reasons for it. If they leave guilt aside, and relax about the relationship, they may perhaps discover that the love that bonded them is still there.'

You have to recalibrate for long-term love, in other words. In Anthony Marra's collection of stories *The Tsar of Love and Techno* (2017), one woman thinks of how 'she'd imagined love to be a flare sparkling upward, unzipping the night sky. What she had with the Russian gave off a warmth nearer to friendship. That was fine with her. Better the dim heat of a hand in yours than all the fire in the sky . . . They were building a life of small kindnesses together. Some days it was extraordinary.' I'll take that.

We also need to understand that periods in which there is more or less connection are entirely normal in a relationship, and not a sign of anything terminal. The psychotherapist Charlotte Fox Weber, author of *What We Want: A Journey Through Twelve of Our Deepest Desires* (2022), advises that we 'normalise and expect some disconnection in pretty much all relationships, no matter how loving. As human as it is to turn towards each other, it's human to turn away from each other at times. The point is that it is not a sign of some unavoidable tragic fate. It's a signal to take care of your relationship.' If you reconnect there can be more joy. 'When we reconnect, we can discover new things about each other and ourselves; this is how we grow.'

Clichés are often clichés for a reason. So here's the ultimate one: the idea that opposites attract. In *The Successful Self* (1988) Dorothy Rowe, who was 56 at the time, declared that 'so far, and my researches among family, friends, clients and acquaintances extend over many years and many couples, I have not come across a couple made up of two introverts or two extraverts. I have met couples who thought they were two introverts, but who, when they considered it, realised that one of them was a shy extravert, or an extravert with a passionate interest in his or her internal reality. I have met extraverts who thought that their partner was also an extravert, but was in fact a socially skilled introvert.'

To be clear, Rowe's definitions of these two personality types are not quite the same as those used in common parlance, but rather as they appeared earlier in the work of Carl Jung, among others. They refer not so much to how you interact with other people as to how you experience the world. You can be a socially adept introvert, or a less socially motivated extravert. The distinction lies in which you see as your stronger reality, your interior life or the world exterior to you. This in turn shapes both what gives your life meaning, and what you perceive as an existential threat.

For Rowe, an extravert is someone who experiences

their existence 'as being a member of a group, as the relationship, the connection, between yourself and others'. An introvert, on the other hand, experiences it 'as the progressive development of your individuality in terms of clarity, achievement and authenticity'.

We are drawn to our opposite in romantic relationships, Rowe argues, because they cement our sense of reality by strengthening the realm that is weakest for us. But if we aren't careful, that complementary way of seeing the world which first bonded us can be an oppositional approach that pulls us apart. To continue to value each other's differences, as we did in the earliest days, months and years of our relationship, rather than to resent them and/or feel alienated by them, is another secret to long-term love.

The American psychologist John Gottman says that it's not difference that is the death knell to a relationship but how we navigate it. It's not even about the degree to which a couple does or doesn't argue, but about how it resolves any such disagreement.

A famous longitudinal experiment by Gottman and Robert Levenson, a psycho-physiologist, comprised interviews with couples about all aspects of their relationship and lives which took place over the course of many years. 'To our surprise,' says Gottman, 'we found that if we had three hours with a couple, we were able to predict with around 90% accuracy which couples would stay together, and which would get divorced, as well as how happy they would be together.' By far and away the best predictor, the researchers determined, was the presence of contempt. 'In good relationships, the level of contempt is almost zero. If they do say something that's regrettable and insulting to their partner, they tend to apologise and repair.'

There are absences that can be almost as telling. A couple that laughs together stays together. You need to have a sense of humour and a sense of fun. Both of which – together with shared and separate passions – will bring you joy as a couple, and joy, as we have already discussed, is where it is at.

Another warning sign that Gottman and Levenson pinpointed after 14 years of data was not contemptuousness but emotional detachment. These were couples who – typically after around 16 years of marriage – 'were leading parallel lives,' according to Gottman. 'And the best indicator that we found was the absence of any positive emotion. There was no affection or interest in each other, or shared humour.'

Of course it can be hard to stay connected, never mind to find time for fun, when you have been together for a while and/or are facing such pressures as child-rearing. If necessary you may – ridiculous as it sounds – need to schedule in some fun, if not some downright silliness. Perhaps this entails doing a new activity together. It might equally be revisiting something you used to do in the early days of your time together.

The psychotherapist Philippa Perry observes in Natasha Lunn's *Conversations in Love* (2021) that the most common roles in a relationship are 'the dreamer' and 'the accountant', and that each partner normally takes one of those roles. She suggests that partners actively take turns. Sex is another element that, after a while, may need some scheduling, not to mention rethinking.

The marital therapist Andrew G Marshall identifies three different sexual phases in the typical relationship.

In the earliest days it's about spontaneous sex which is 'driven by novelty' and 'can help you to get to know each other better'. The next phase is validation sex, when you are starting really to care about each other and each wants validation and reassurance from the other that they feel the same way. This, however, is when things can start to go a bit wrong. Life might be getting in the way, be it young children or other stresses and strains.

'Women can start responding to their husband's desire – rather than feeling their own – and have sex to please him or start to fake their response. Men may be aware their wife is exhausted from work and childcare so become more inclined to cut right to the chase, rather than focus on her pleasure. Both partners can end up feeling more an object than validated.' What I would add is that I think many women, whether they realise it or not, start to feel underserved by the sexual act. Quite simply, it isn't pushing their buttons any more, or ringing their bells. More on this in a minute.

The key, says Marshall, is to find your way to what he calls connection sex. 'This is where you bring all of yourself to the bedroom and take the risk of opening up to your partner about your desires – which are probably very different from when you first met. Far more than that spontaneous first kind, and objectifying second, it's Connection Sex [Marshall's capitalisation] that has the potential to keep on getting better and better.'

And of course as we learn to connect more with ourselves, through ageing consciously and wisely, and being more honest about that self, its needs and desires, we have a greater chance at connection sex. Forty per cent of the people interviewed for the book *Magnificent Sex: Lessons from Extraordinary Lovers* (2020), co-authored by Peggy Kleinplatz, a professor of medicine and a sex researcher, and Dana Ménard, a psychology professor, were in their sixties, seventies and eighties. One commonality was that they had a better sense of what they wanted as they aged, and were more willing to articulate it. They were also more willing to express vulnerability. Another was that they spoke of the idea of 'embodiment'. As one man put it, 'You are not the person in the situation. You *are* it. You *are* the situation.'

Another book that – alongside Fromm's *Art of Loving* – I believe should be part of everyone's arsenal is *Love, Freedom, Aloneness* (2001) by the controversial spiritual teacher Osho. That's especially the case if you are single. Admittedly you might want to park memories of Netflix's documentary *Wild Wild Country* (2018) should you have seen it, which depicts the late guru as not without his foibles, 93 of which came in the form of Rolls-Royces gifted to him by his followers. His words, however, are unquestionably wise and useful, especially if you are retooling yourself after the end of a relationship and/or are wanting a road map for singledom that is as far removed from spinsterdom as it is possible to get.

Here's Osho on the joy of aloneness: 'The moment you feel you are no longer dependent on anyone, a deep coolness and a deep silence settles inside, a relaxed let-go. It does not mean you stop loving. On the contrary, for the first time you know a new quality, a new dimension of love – a love that is no longer biological, a love that is closer to friendliness than any relationship.'

And here is Osho on relationships, or rather, as he assiduously differentiates, relating: 'Love is never a relationship; love is relating. It is always a river, flowing, unending . . . It is an ongoing phenomenon. Lovers end, love continues – it is a continuum. It is a verb, not a noun . . .' (Echoes of Fromm.)

'Hence I say relate,' he continues. 'By saying relate, I mean remain continuously on a honeymoon. Go on searching and seeking each other, finding new ways of loving each other, finding new ways of being with each other. And each person is such an infinite mystery, inexhaustible, unfathomable, that it is not possible you can ever say, "I have known her," or "I have known him." At the most you can say, "I have tried my best, but the mystery remains a mystery." In fact the more you know, the more mysterious the other becomes. Then love is a constant adventure.'

And here, finally, is Osho rebutting the idea that we must be in one camp or the other, either fully signed up to life in a couple or to a life alone, but can instead be led only by what – and who – is right for us as we are today: 'It is beautiful to be alone; it is also beautiful to be in love. And they are complementary, not contradictory. When you are enjoying others, enjoy, and enjoy to the fullest; there is no need to bother about aloneness. And when you are fed up with others, then move into aloneness and enjoy it to the fullest.'

The end of a relationship is never a disaster, even if it wasn't your choice. It is an opportunity. We are taught to see an ending as failure, as an unfortunate erasure of the happy-ever-after we have been programmed to believe in since we were children. We are taught that an ending negates the relationship that preceded it pretty much in its entirety.

Why should this be the case? It is always the right and brave thing to do to pursue love. As the 13th-century Persian poet Rumi put it:

Someone who does not run
toward the allure of love
walks a road where nothing lives.

Dr Habib Sadeghi takes a rather more medical approach to the power of love, pointing out that 'the bioelectromagnetic field of the heart is 5,000 times stronger than the brain', and asks who wouldn't want to channel some of that?

Yet it is also the right and brave thing to do to move on from a relationship when it no longer serves. There are countless other ways to find and experience love and connectedness. Seeking out a new partner may not even be the best way to do it. It is loving and connecting with yourself that is most important.

I see my own past relationships as chapters in the book of me, the ending of each one a caesura, not a stop, and the very thing that facilitated the beginning of something else, by which I don't necessarily mean another relationship, but a period of self-growth. Each one made me happy for as long as it made me happy, and each one taught me a huge amount even – especially – after it stopped making me happy.

I would agree with Andrew G Marshall that spending a year or two single after the end of a significant relationship is a good idea. 'We make the mistake of expecting to recover too quickly from the break-up of an important relationship,' he writes. 'It normally takes 18 months to two years to move on, and, unless you give yourself time to learn the lessons from one relationship, you will take them into your next.'

If and when you are ready to meet someone – and, to reiterate, it's an entirely valid choice to have no interest in doing so, whether that's for now or forever – the apps are waiting for you. I can't pretend that it doesn't pain me just a little to have to write that sentence, because I know how bruising they can be, and how strange. I think it's a loss for us all that real-world flirtation has become so rare. But apps can work.

What we needed was a proper recalibration of real-world flirtation and dating, not an out-and-out stoppage. We needed men still to chat women up, but in an appropriate way, interested rather than leerily, with an understanding that 'no' means no. And we needed women to feel empowered to chat men up just as much. But that hasn't happened. The entire activity has pretty much died out.

We are also dealing with the diminution of those previously discussed bridging groups in favour of the stronger connections of bonded groups. The latter is made up of people like us, and is exclusive. A bridging group is inclusive, and open to anyone who is prepared to abide by its rules.

'Bonding groups are good for getting by,' says Marshall, who offers workshops on finding love. 'Intimate friends rally round when we are in trouble. But bridging capital is vital for getting on. This is because acquaintances are more likely to provide a lead for a new job, or, more important for single people, an introduction to a potential partner.'

To actively seek out bridging groups is one way to open yourself to the possibility of meeting someone. You need new people to be crossing your path regularly. A friend of mine who has been single for years has transformed his friendship group recently by signing up for a weekly streetdance class, and by working one shift a week in a bar that's full of creative people of all ages whom he finds inspiring. Will it transform his romantic life? Time will tell. Meanwhile, at least as importantly, he is having a wonderful time. You need to make an effort to meet new people, whether your end goal is to find a 'someone' or just to have a more full and varied life.

I know how counterintuitive it can be for many older women to put themselves on the apps in the first place. The very act of advertising yourself seems somehow unladylike, desperate or both. I felt the same myself when I first joined them. It's a totally quotidian thing to do these days, however, and I think that if you do want to meet someone, you would be missing a trick not to give it a go. Ultimately it worked for me.

Meeting the right person, someone who really fits, is as much as anything else a numbers game. And in the real world the numbers just aren't that great. The apps change that. Until recently a divorcee or a widow might never meet anyone again, or might feel she had to settle for pretty much any single man to cross her path. Not any more. A friend who is a facialist once told me that for decades her female clients would lie on her couch lamenting how impossible it was to meet anyone. 'No one does that any more,' she laughs. These days we may lament the slings and arrows of the apps – I know I have! – but meeting people is the easiest it has ever been.

I am not saying it is going to be straightforward. You need to set yourself a few guidelines before you start.

You also need to understand that it might be a bumpy road at times. But it *is* a road. If you do it in the right way it will take you somewhere, even if that somewhere isn't necessarily a relationship but some new learning about yourself and the world.

The American journalist and screenwriter Nora Ephron's mantra was 'Everything is copy.' This was the woman who turned a miserable divorce – her husband cheated on her when she was pregnant – into *Heartburn* (1983), one of the funniest books ever written. I think this is a great approach when it comes to dating, if not to life in general. You don't need to be a writer to see that everything and everyone can be a story, an anecdote waiting to be told. It might be funny, or it might be terrible (and also, after time, and with the right attitude, funny), and it may well have some learning wrapped up in it somewhere.

I treated my dates like a kind of assignment, meeting people I would usually never have come across otherwise, and setting out to find out what it is like to, say, be in the army or grow up in Jamaica. I kept things short (a coffee or a drink; no one can become boring that quickly if you ask the right questions). And I was similarly disciplined about the time I dedicated to the apps when I wasn't actually on a date.

The trick is that you need to check in regularly – consistency is key if you want to meet the best people – but not for very long. And you need to banish it from your mind for the rest of the time. What happens to many people is that they become obsessive and, ultimately, addicted. The apps are wired for precisely that to happen. Demarcate 20 to 30 minutes once a day, at a time that best helps you put it in a metaphorical box and close the lid afterwards. (That's why I wouldn't advocate it last thing at night.) Set an alarm. Stop when it goes off.

Equally important is that you keep in your mind that nothing – and no one – is concrete until they prove themselves in the real world, and over time. The apps are full of lost souls, confused men and women who say one thing and do another; who think they want one thing – perhaps you – and then don't. Don't make any assumptions at all until you meet someone. And still don't make any assumptions even then. Even supposed adults behave like adolescent flibbertigibbets on the apps. I met one apparent grown-up – a KC in his fifties – who was telling me that he loved me within weeks. (On our first date he told me he couldn't wait for me to meet his mother. Admittedly a bad sign in retrospect!) Weeks after that he had ghosted me. Brilliantly he once sent me a WhatsApp telling me that he was 'faking [sic] in love' with me. Turns out that faking it was precisely what he was doing! As I said, everything is copy.

What's key is to remain open but protected, vulnerable yet impermeable, an apparently contradictory state that it can be difficult to maintain but that is a fantastic way to approach so many aspects of life. I know people who have left themselves so open as to be profoundly hurt. I know others who have protected themselves so much that, whether they are on the apps or not, their heart is too armour-plated to allow for love.

It was the invention of the pill that enabled the modern incarnation of dating, predicated as it is not just on plenty-of-sex-before-marriage but, often as not, on sex-after-date-two. The argument has often been made that it is women, the supposed winners when it comes to female contraception, who have ended up losing out. The fact that, once upon a time, a nice girl didn't, meant that a nice boy had to commit to a relationship of some kind in order to be able to sleep with her.

That now – in the West at least – women are as sexually liberated as men – in theory at least – is, of course, a good thing. However, the tyranny of choice, which in turn leads to the tyranny of non-commitment, means that many young people, men as well as women, are finding it difficult even to have a proper relationship, never mind to find a good one. The apps are the ultimate manifestation of that, and in theory the ultimate male dream. But men are increasingly hoist by their own petard. My partner's assorted male confidants in their twenties and thirties are – after years of dating – as battle-weary and wary as the women I know of the same age.

Then there's the sex. The modern dating scene is largely based on the idea that more is more, in the sense of both the number of partners you have, and the amount of sex. Our idea of a good sex life has been cobbled together from largely benign pantomimes such as *Sex and the City* and the far from benign behemoth which is the porn industry. Almost everywhere we look, to a degree that most of us don't realise, it remains a male envisioning of sex, not a female one. Even *Sex and the City* was written by a man.

Sex has become the ultimate act of doing, rather than being; an act, not a state. Even the term 'making love' – a turn of phrase that encapsulates both an emotional and a creative dimension – has come to seem old-fashioned. The apps take matters further, turning the search for connection into a kind of shopping; into sexual consumerism. Certainly we needed some kind of sexual revolution – after centuries when women were discouraged from embracing their sexuality, and judged if they didn't conform – but we have gone too far, or rather, we have gone in the wrong direction.

Sharon Olds's poem 'Sex without Love' (1984) is a provocative meditation on how having sex – however good that sex may superficially be – differs from the more profound act of making love. I urge you to look it up if you don't know it. What she describes is an encounter that is as much disconnection as connection. In my experience, however good it might be in the moment, sex without love can be a discombobulating, even a deracinating experience.

One of the most eye-opening – not to mention game-changing – books I have ever read is Diana Richardson's *Tantric Orgasm for Women* (2004). It's easy to get put off by words like Tantra. Whose mind doesn't immediately jump to those long-ago Sting anecdotes – part hilarious, part terrifying – of how he and his wife liked to have Tantric sex for hours?! In fact, it's a simple concept based around the idea of intercourse as an exchange of different energies between a man and a woman, and of making love as a state in which you reside without particular focus or effort rather than a goal-oriented – for which read orgasm-driven – act. It is more about being than doing, once again.

It helps to explain why making love with someone you care about and who cares about you can have a dimension to it that's not as easily found in a different sort of encounter. It helps to explain why even the most fantastic one-night stand can offer up, alongside the ecstasy, a more enduring kind of emptiness. It helps to explain why many women start to go off sex after they have been with the same partner for some time. Put bluntly, the thrusting that tends to be seen as a key part of sex, at least among heterosexuals, is just not doing it for them any more.

Should you choose to follow some of Tantra's teaching, even if only some of the time, it may help you to find your way to the best sex of your life. This is the ultimate connection sex, and it – like you – can get better with age.

11

Working It

Does your work feel like play to you, or like work, somewhere on the scale of mildly taxing to downright onerous? Or does it feel like something else again, an abnegation of who you are?

Perhaps your job used to feel like you, like fun even, and now it doesn't. It can be hard to maintain your enthusiasm and energy levels over the many decades that typically equate to a working life. What's more, in a society that skews towards ageism, the workplace is another sphere in which you can start to feel invisible: overlooked and unheard.

How best to navigate the workplace as you get older? How best to navigate leaving the workplace when you retire? That's what I am going to look at in this chapter. My focus, in truth, will be as much on not working as on working. This is because I believe that cultural conditioning encourages everyone – or at least everyone lucky enough through upbringing and education to have professional aspirations in the first place – to put too much weight on their work as the source of their identity.

It is also because many of us women find ourselves, whether by choice or necessity, taking a step back professionally after we have children. This is not the place to go into the unfairness of many working mothers' position in the workplace, but it is the place to look at what work isn't, as well as what it is.

For me 'working it' in the fullest sense is about calibrating all the different aspects of your existence so that together they give you the means to be the best you yet. That may in fact equate to working less. Or it may involve making your peace with the irresolvable frustrations and limitations of your job, the better to leave you the time and the headspace to expand in other areas of your life.

We are encouraged to believe that our job defines us; that it is one of the most important things about us. And we are encouraged – nay, expected – to put the hours in accordingly. Albert Schweitzer put this – like much else he considered negative about the modern human experience – at the door of the Industrial Revolution. 'For two or three generations many individuals have lived only as working beings, not as human beings,' he wrote in the 1920s. We are human beings. Or at least we should be. We aren't what we do for a living. It may be a part of who we are, but it is only a part, and we need to find more manifold ways to build our identity.

Luckily as women we tend to have a head start in this regard. Motherhood may mean that we have faced workplace discrimination, whether it's explicit or stems from the impossibility of keeping all the balls in the air. (Society has such a long way to go when it comes to understanding that childcare, to name but one issue, is a collective problem, not one that can legitimately be left to individuals.) Yet it also accustomises us to seeing ourselves in different ways and different arenas, and for other people to view us similarly. That's the case even for women who, like me, haven't actually had children themselves.

As yet men tend to be more straitjacketed into old-fashioned conceptions about being the provider. This means it can be less easy for them to shapeshift, whether that's professionally or in other ways, and they can struggle more with doing a job that isn't enough for them in some way. It's an aside, but a fascinating one, the degree to which the male identity still tends to be more wrapped up in what they do – or don't do – for a living than the female. Certainly it is something that more than one ex-partner of mine has struggled with to a degree that I haven't found among my girlfriends.

In her thought-provoking book-cum-treatise *For The Love of Men: A New Vision of Mindful Masculinity* (2019), the American journalist Liz Plank writes of how society still expects men to foot the bill, whether that's literal or metaphorical, and how this expectation doesn't serve either men or women well. By way of one example, Plank, a fellow dating-apps survivor, writes about how, like me, she has been gobsmacked by the continued 'collective insistence on one gender paying for the other gender as an ultimate sign of respect'.

What might seem a passing detail is deeply revealing about how men are still brought up to see themselves, and their role in the world. Set that alongside another message men now receive, namely that women want to be treated as equals, and men are, Plank says, 'justifiably lost'. This is compelling stuff, but I digress. What is relevant here is that it continues to be easier for women to choose *not* to identify with what they do for a living. Many men don't feel as if they have that luxury.

In the 1970s, the Pulitzer-Prize-winning historian Studs Terkel spoke to dozens of pseudonymous workers across America – from a professor to a cab driver – for his now famous book of reportage called *Working: People Talk About What They Do All Day and How They Feel About What They Do* (1974). What was one take-away from Terkel's masterpiece? 'Most of us . . . have jobs that are too small for our spirit,' one of his interviewees told him. 'Jobs are not big enough for people.'

However, Terkel also documented the way people found succour in doing their job well, whatever it was and however mundane it might be. 'Dolores Dante graphically describes the trials of a waitress in a fashionable restaurant,' he writes in his introduction. 'They are compounded by her refusal to be demeaned. Yet pride in her skills helps her make it through the night. 'When I put the plate down, you don't hear a sound. When I pick up a glass, I want it to be just right. When someone says, "How come you're just a waitress?" I say, "Don't you think you deserve being served by me?"''

Terkel characterises his book as being about 'a search . . . for daily meaning as well as daily bread, for recognition as well as cash, for astonishment rather than torpor. In short, for a sort of life rather than a Monday through Friday sort of dying.'

Astonishment. That's such a big word, a big feeling. It's a lot to ask of many jobs. However, astonishment or, at the very least, interest, is everywhere if we just look for it. It reminds me of another of my favourite Mary Oliver quotes, from her poem 'Sometimes':

Instructions for living a life:

Pay attention.

Be astonished.

Tell about it.

Some of us will succeed at that in our work, and some will fail. But that's OK. We can feed our spirit in other ways. We may be lucky enough to be able to expand our professional life so that it reflects more of who we really feel ourselves to be. Yet if that option isn't open to us, then we can deepen and broaden our experience of being alive through other means, and we can also find import, like Dolores Dante, in the way we put down a plate or pick up a glass, or whatever our equivalent may be. That, after all, is what most of our ancestors had to do, until the large-scale social mobility of the last century transformed mainstream expectations around work.

My grandfather left school at 13 and was apprenticed to a builder. Construction was what he did until the day he retired. But what he loved – was truly passionate about – was art. He filled his spare time with painting, along with gardening, hill-walking and what I like to call gourmandising – he loved food and wine. There was nothing wrong with what he did for a living. He didn't dislike it. But nor did he expect it to define him.

This is something that many of us have lost. How fortunate we are, in most ways, that this is the case. What a privilege it is – a privilege my grandfather would have embraced – to have the opportunity to find a job that you feel fulfils you, encapsulates you even. However, those jobs will always be few and far between, much more so than modern narratives around work would suggest.

That Elizabeth Jane Howard quote in the last chapter about the supposed abundance of that incredibly elusive phenomenon, a deep and enduring love match, could, I believe, be as easily applied to the workplace. Just as many of us tire of a partner who, at the beginning, seemed like the right person for us, and yet still continue to go through the motions, many of us stay in a job when we know it is past its sell-by date or, at the very least, doesn't excite us and/or fulfil us in the way it once did. Why? Because it pays the bills, of course. And because finding something else can feel at best difficult, at worst impossible.

I happen to think that can be all right. As long, that is, as you have other passions that excite and fulfil you in your life. I believe my grandfather's blueprint for work remains a valid one. As for his move into retirement, that, if anything, entailed an increase in activity. Certainly it was a diversification. I still remember as a little girl watching his vast builder's hands, elegant but exhausted-looking, laminating his croissant dough on the kitchen table. Baking was just one of the hobbies Grandad Walter got into in his seventies.

In recent years I have met a new group of people who have chosen to organise their lives more along his lines, albeit perhaps in more 21st-century ways. Many of them are friends of my partner's. They are mostly, like him, highly creative. In the first year or so, before I had met many of them, I would hear about one who was an artist, another who was a drummer, and so it went on. It was only gradually that I began to discover that they earn a living in other ways entirely. They have perfectly good jobs, but those jobs are not who they are.

Now that I have met them, I know them to be some of the most contented, not to mention dynamic, people

I have ever come across. They are full of ambitions, but those ambitions are not necessarily connected to what they do for a living. They are about a piece of music they are composing, or a canvas they are painting, or a skateboarding trick that – in their sixties! – they are still finessing.

Your actual job may be something that you need to dial down, in terms of the effort and/or headspace it takes up, in order for you to be able to live more fully. In China a phenomenon known as #tangping or 'lying flat' has taken root among young people. It's the antithesis of Sheryl Sandberg's 'lean in' mantra, in other words, in which you do more, push more, and focus on an upward trajectory, very possibly – as her phraseology inadvertently signals – at the cost of living in balance. In the West it has come to be known as 'quiet quitting'. You do your job. You don't let your job do you.

This, for me, is working it. It is also the perfect way to ease yourself into life after work. What do those friends of my other half's take home at the end of every month? Money to settle their bills, certainly. But also the best riches of all: living in joy. If your job doesn't fulfil you or express you, and you can't find your way to one that does, find your joy elsewhere.

Let's move on to some practical advice about the workplace now. Whether you experience your job as a means to self-realisation or simply to pay off the mortgage, there are ways to render yourself more visible; there are ways to become more 'you'. Let's consider what can be done to surface yourself; to mitigate against being sidelined or discriminated against because you happen not to be 28 any more.

I won't presume to tell you how to do the nitty-gritty of your job well, not least because I don't know what you do for a living. What I will say is that how you show up, in terms of the way you do what you do, and the way you look while you are doing it, can be game-changers.

Let's start with the way you present yourself. To reiterate, I am a huge believer in the power of clothes to transform the way others see you, and there is no context in which this can have more traction than at work. Work dressing is the most codified around. You and your cohort form a tribe, whether you like it or not, and one of the ways a tribe bonds is through dress.

Go the full David Attenborough on your tribe. With fresh eyes, study what similarities there are around how people dress. What do they wear or not wear? Even in the most supposedly non-conformist working environment there will be a uniform or uniforms in play.

I would argue that you want to fit in to some degree, but that you want to stand out, too. Getting noticed in the right way can give you power. Even – especially – if yours is a conventionally smart environment, you need to be wary of being too conformist. You also want to be careful about personifying clichéd notions of how an older woman looks and dresses. Overly smart can appear dated, and to appear dated – it goes without saying – is one of the most ageing things you can do.

Do you have any colleagues who are surfacing themselves sartorially in a way that works, anyone you can learn from? Take notes. Think too about that word you came up with in Chapter 8. Does it apply to you in a professional capacity? As I said before, I would argue that, like my word 'interesting', it ideally should. I would also argue that, if you can't find a word that feels relevant to both your personal and professional personas, there is a disconnect there that might be indicative of a bigger problem.

It's not that 'interesting' has to mean the same in the two contexts, for example, but that it can be redeployed in both. That said, if you are insistent that you need two words – and, given that a number of my friends are, I feel I have to give you a pass on this! – then pin down your second one. Is your current work wardrobe successfully communicating this to everyone else?

If you spend a lot of your job at your desk and/or on Zoom, being seen from the waist up, you should finesse a particular sartorial skillset known as above-the-desk dressing. Make sure you get that bit of you right. A great pair of earrings and/or a necklace can be enough to lift an otherwise straight-down-the-line ensemble. As discussed, I love modernised pearls, especially in the workplace, because they not only flatter the complexion, just as our grandmothers' were designed to do, but also subtly contemporise your look. That popping lipstick or a strong eye we have already talked about can be similarly transformative.

Don't underestimate the power of colour and pattern, be it on a blouse layered under a dark suit or indeed the suit itself. Suits and dresses are the simplest way to present as pulled together, given that they do most of the work for you of a morning. A jumpsuit pulls off the same trick, and reliably comes off as bang up to date. These days you can even buy pinstriped ones. A woman in a jumpsuit comes across as someone who is open and youthful in her approach. Now, with the right jumpsuit, she can signal that she is a professional, too. If the idea still doesn't appeal, just think of it as another kind of dress, albeit one that comes with legs!

Remember too that shoes are one of the easiest ways to carbon-date someone. Keeping your footwear choices current will make you appear current, and appearing current means you are more likely to be assumed to *be* current. An athleisure reference here and there can sprinkle similar magic dust, whether you pair your suit with a fresh white T-shirt, or perhaps go for a dress or tailoring with zip or elastication detailing.

Does this all seem superficial to you? Can I remind

you of the charity Smart Works that I mentioned in Chapter 8? It was the moment when the women saw themselves for the first time in a professional-looking get-up that they were fully able to envisage themselves as someone who had the capacity to secure a job.

The social psychologist Amy Cuddy talks about what she calls the 'power pose', in which people who adopt an open and expansive stance to make themselves appear bigger than they are feel more powerful as a result, and are interpreted as such by others. I believe clothes can be a power pose of their own.

I imagine that, like me, you had some intimation of this if you had to work from home during the pandemic. Did you bother to dress properly for work in the first few weeks? I know I didn't. How did that make you feel? How well did that make you do your job? I would place money on the fact that, like me, your sense of purpose and professionalism was transformed when you started to dress the part again, or at least an approximation of the part that felt right when working from your kitchen table or spare bedroom.

What the pandemic also underlined – whether it's for

workwear or anything else – is that being comfortable is a no-brainer. It's not only a needless waste of headspace to be uncomfortable – the world is thankfully these days full of clothes that are as cool and chic as they are comfy – it's also, and I am going to use that 'd' word again, dating to look as if you aren't relaxed in what you are wearing. You want footwear you can walk in, clothes that don't require you to hold your breath.

All of these elements will help you to be taken on your own merits in the workplace. But so too, if you deploy it adroitly, will the wisdom you have built up over years. Whatever changes in the workplace, whether that's down to technology or anything else, there's one constant: people. And you – as you continue to do the work on yourself, and to treat the act of living as a learning experience, as an accumulation rather than a depletion – will have understanding and insights that others younger than you, not to mention those of a similar vintage, may not.

It's all about how you share your learning. No one likes a know-it-all. Besides, if you have properly been working on yourself, if anything you will be more in touch with what you still have to learn than what you already have.

It's also about a two-way street; about those very same skills we deploy in our personal relationships. Being as much – if not more – a listener as a speaker. Sharing ideas and suggestions, rather than supposed rights and supposed wrongs.

Anyone with any sense knows that there is nothing more precious than to come across someone clued up and compassionate who is further down the line than them in the same game, whether said game pertains to their chosen profession or life as a whole. Make yourself that person. Speak your truth, but always calmly and compassionately. See your job not just as your job, but as a way of serving others; of making their jobs – and, as a result, their lives – better.

I have spoken to a number of friends considerably younger than me about their conceptions of the older people at their work. They have told me how much they relish the presence of those older colleagues they consider to offer the best combination of experience and openness. These are people who demonstrate that neurological aptitude that Daniel Levitin calls 'generalisation' in tandem, as per M Scott Peck, with the desire to keep making new maps. One friend has told me about the sense of 'stability' and 'wisdom' one particular man in his sixties brings to any working group at their offices, and how everyone feels better when that individual is involved. 'Unlike so many of the younger ones, he doesn't have a personal agenda. He isn't driven by ego. He just wants to make the group as a whole, and us as individuals, better at what we are doing.'

Through your work – as through every other kind of human connection in your life – you have the chance to help others; to model a way of being in the world that they may not have been shown before. Ralph Waldo Emerson wrote, 'To leave the world a bit better, whether by a healthy child, a garden patch, or a redeemed social condition; to know that even one life has breathed easier because you have lived – that is to have succeeded.' To offer a colleague or three guidance and compassion, better still to point them in the direction of their road less travelled, also equates to success.

Because actually it is not what you do but, once

again, how you do it. To revisit that Pema Chödrön quote, 'Everything in our lives can wake us up or put us to sleep, and basically it's up to us to let it wake us up.' And that includes work, even at its most apparently banal. Not every workplace will offer up the bandwidth required for you to make structural change around you, but you can always change – and improve – yourself, whether it is in how you go about your tasks or in how you interact.

There is a woman who works at my local supermarket who is one of the sunniest people I have ever come across. Mainly her job is loitering around the self check-out helping shoppers with all those petty problems that annoyingly seem to crop up when you are left to swipe your own groceries. But what she also does is smile a lot and say jolly things. I once wrote about her in *The Times*, and how much – although I didn't even know her name – she meant to me. Numerous people got in touch to say that she meant something to them, too.

The pandemic shed light on the bogus hierarchy of jobs, underlining the fact that we need supermarket workers and dustbin men as well as mortgage brokers and high-court judges. That woman's job has value in that she helps get food to our tables. Without her, and the millions of other workers in the food industry, the supply chain would soon break down. But she has made her job important in another way because of how she does it. A supposedly humdrum role has become, courtesy of what she puts into it, an activity that changes a wide range of lives for the better.

She isn't leaning in in the Sandberg sense; nor is she lying down. Rather she is holding her space, helping others, as a human being who happens to work, not a working being who happens to be human. She is one of those 'hidden' people George Eliot wrote of. She's not going to make the obituary pages; in this regard hers will be one of the 'unvisited tombs'. Yet it is in part because of her 'unhistoric acts' – along with those of many millions of others – that the 'growing good of the world' depends. As I get older, that for me has become what working it is really about.

12

Destination You

What an amazing gift, the gift of ageing. There is no period of life better calibrated for making friends with the real you. You have more data to go on, but you also have the wisdom to let go of the data; to be in the moment, or – to put it more simply still – to be.

That in itself explains why old age is so discomfiting a state for many. Eckhart Tolle encapsulates the issue perfectly in *A New Earth: Awakening to Your Life's Purpose* (2005). 'Why is old considered useless? Because in old age, the emphasis shifts from doing to Being, and our civilization, which is lost in doing, knows nothing of Being. It asks: Being? What do you do with it?'

What do you do with it? You find your true self – the

most fully realised, fully expanded version you have uncovered to date. Ipseity, the state of selfhood, is your goal. Nothing less. What joy and what richness that will bring to you. And just by being that self, you will, whether consciously or unconsciously, bring joy and richness to others.

There is a Sudanese proverb that says, 'We desire to bequeath two things to our children; the first one is roots, the other one is wings.' For most of us it is in fact only when we move towards old age that we start to develop the wisdom that will enable us to turn that apparent contradiction into our reality. Wings and roots. We can grow them both.

I hope this little book of what I have learned so far may help you a bit with both the wings and the roots; may ease your path towards a deeper understanding of another dichotomy. Because, as W B Yeats wrote in 'Sailing to Byzantium':

An aged man is but a paltry thing,
A tattered coat upon a stick, unless
Soul clap its hands and sing, and louder sing . . .

Here's to our soul clapping its hands and singing; more than that, to it dancing, laughing and eating cake, plus maybe, in my case at least, finally pulling off an unsupported handstand!

I am sure there is much that I should have said in this book and haven't. There is certainly at least another book's worth to be written on what I haven't yet learned. Perhaps I will write that one when I am 80, when there will again be one more shadow book that exists alongside it containing all that about which I continue to be ignorant.

Elizabeth Jane Howard was 79 when she wrote her memoir *Slipstream* (2002). In its final pages she sums up what she had found out thus far – what she is continuing to find out – about ageing. Howard is typically honest, not to mention sage, in her taking stock.

'It's clear to me now that inside the conspiracy of silence about age – because of the negative aspects of the condition – there is the possibility of art; that is to say that it can be made into something worth trying to do well, a challenge, an adventure,' she writes. 'I want to live inquiringly, with curiosity and interest for the rest of my life.'

'The possibility of art.' 'A challenge, an adventure.' Yes, to all this. And yes to living 'inquiringly, with curiosity and interest'. I hope this book has inspired you to feel similarly about the years ahead; to feel excited, and engaged, and also brave about whatever the future holds. In 'A Poet's Advice to Students' (*A Miscellany*, 1958), E E Cummings advocated being 'nobody-but-yourself', an act that 'in a world which is doing its best, night and day to make you everybody else – means to fight the hardest battle which any human being can fight; and never stop fighting'. This isn't at all 'dismal', he goes on to insist. 'It's the most wonderful life on earth.'

Cummings may have been talking to would-be poets. I think his words apply to all of us. And that this is a wonderful life indeed. What's more, I believe it can grow more wonderful as we grow older. I believe that with age that 'fight' he writes about can transform into more of a dance: light and joyful and *fun*. A dance. A glorious dance to the death.

Notes

Chapter 1   What's Gone Wrong, and How to Make It Right

21 *'Keep some room in your heart*   From the collection *Evidence: Poems* by Mary Oliver (Beacon Press, Boston, 2009).

Chapter 2   Finding Your Purpose

25 *As the Buddhist nun*   Robina Courtin quote posted on Instagram on 14 November 2021.

28 *In his book*   Published as *Successful Aging: A Neuroscientist Explores the Power and Potential of Our Lives* in the USA (Dutton, New York, 2020).

30 *Or, as the 13th-century theologian*   *Meister Eckhart: A Modern Translation* by Raymond B Blakney (Harper & Row, New York, 1941).

36 *Someone I loved*   From the collection *Thirst: Poems by Mary Oliver* (Beacon Press, Boston, 2006).

Chapter 3 Saying Goodbye, Saying Hello

52 *Dr Max Pemberton*   'Sorry, but midlife horrors aren't just hormonal' by Dr Max Pemberton, *Daily Mail*, 23 October 2022.

Chapter 4 How (and Why) to Live in Joy

70 *The Russian literary critic*   As quoted in *The Master and His Emissary: The Divided Brain and the Making of the Western World* by Iain McGilchrist (Yale University Press, 2009).

89 *As the 20th-century German theologian*   From a letter Schweitzer wrote to his friend Erwin R Jacobi in 1962, as cited in *To Have or to Be?* by Erich Fromm (Harper & Row, New York, 1976).

90 *As the 89-year-old Joan Bakewell*   'Joan Bakewell on affairs, King Charles and her J K Rowling tweet' by Helen Rumbelow, *The Times*, 4 October 2022.

90 *It's not just writers who*   From the introduction to *The Early Stories: 1953–1975* by John Updike (Knopf, New York, 2003).

Chapter 5 Embracing Your Face

102 *'On so many levels it is wrong,'*   'The Lesley Manville Interview: Plastic surgery feels like a betrayal of our sex' by Susannah Butter, London *Evening Standard*, 11 August 2021.

103 *Or as another actress*   'Renée Zellweger: "You've got to survive a lot to get to my age" by Christa D'Souza, *The Times*, 7 August 2022.

103 *And to quote one final actress*   Helena Bonham Carter: Good on young men for finding middle-aged beauty sexy', *The Sunday Times*, 27 November 2022

Chapter 7 Your Body Beautiful

149 *The columnist Janice Turner* 'Calorie counting can be a lifetime's curse' by Janice Turner, *The Times*, 8 April 2022.

Chapter 9 Family, Old and New

216 *As Nikola Tesla, the Serbian-American inventor* As quoted in *Within: A Spiritual Awakening to Love & Weight Loss* by Dr Habib Sadeghi (Open Road Media, New York, 2013).

223 *'The only sumptom of empty-nest syndrome,'* 'Having children is a joy but it doesn't make us happier' by Emma Duncan, *The Times*, 5 August 2022.

Chapter 10 True Romance

241 *'By finding novelty every day* 'What falling in love does to your mind and body' by Hilary Rose, *The Times*, 14 April 2022.

245 *'In good relationships, the level* 'Physiological and affective predictors of change in relationship satisfaction' by Robert W Levenson, Indiana University, and John M Gottman, University of Illinois, *Journal of Personality and Social Psychology*, 1985, Vol. 49, No. 1, pp. 85–94.

246 *The marital therapist Andrew G Marshall* 'The three types of sex – and why only *one* can put the spark back in your relationship', by Andrew G Marshall, *Daily Mail*, 13 July 2022.

251 *Someone who does not run* From 'The Allure of Love', translated by Coleman Barks, in *Rumi – The Book of Love: Poems of Ecstasy and Longing* (HarperCollins, New York, 2003).

Chapter 11 Working It

265 *'For two or three generations*   From 'Die Schuld der Philosophie an dem Niedergang der Kultur' by Albert Schweitzer (1923), cited by Erich Fromm in *To Have or To Be?* (Harper & Row, New York, 1976).

269 *Instructions for living a life:*   From *Red Bird – Poems by Mary Oliver* (Beacon Press, New York, 2008).

Acknowledgements

'Mattina' taken from *Vita d'un uomo. Tutte le poesie* by
Giuseppe Ungaretti
© 1969 Arnoldo Mondadori Editore S.p.A., Milano
© 2016 Mondadori Libri S.p.A., Milano

'Mindful' by Mary Oliver. Reprinted by the
permission of The Charlotte Sheedy Literary Agency
as agent for the author. Copyright © Mary Oliver
2004, 2005, 2017 with permission of Bill Reichblum

'The Uses of Sorrow' by Mary Oliver. Reprinted by
the permission of The Charlotte Sheedy Literary

Author's Acknowledgements

With thanks to everyone who has helped me find the way to my best me yet. You know who you are. And to my parents. And above all – and always – to Fran.

Index

About the Author

As Fashion Director of *The Times*, it goes without saying that Anna Murphy is passionate about what we wear. The author of *How Not To Wear Black* believes strongly that the supposedly superficial act of choosing what to put on every morning can have a profound impact not just on how we look, but how we feel.

Her years of writing and research, plus her own life experience, have also opened Anna up to fresh thinking around beauty, diet and exercise, and – overarching all of it – the best ways to live a life that is contented and fulfilled, especially as you grow older.

🄰 @annagmurphy

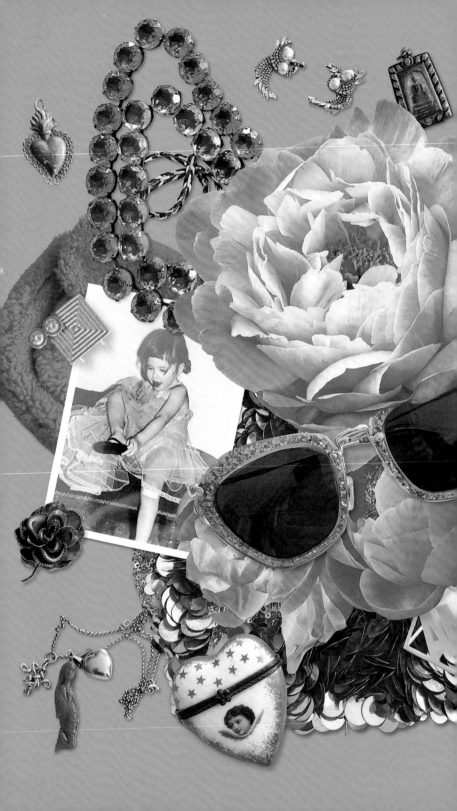